A Path
to Healing

A Path to Healing

A Guide to Wellness for Body, Mind, and Soul

DR. ANDREA D. SULLIVAN

BROADWAY BOOKS

NEW YORK

BROADWAY

A Main Street Books edition of this book was originally published in 1999. It is here reprinted by arrangement with Doubleday.

A Path to Healing. Copyright © 1998 by Andrea D. Sullivan. All rights reserved. Printed in the United States of America. No part of this book may be reproduced or transmitted in any form or by any means, electronic or mechanical, including photocopying, recording, or by any information storage and retrieval system, without written permission from the publisher. For information, address: Broadway Books, a division of Random House, Inc., 1540 Broadway, New York, NY 10036.

Broadway Books titles may be purchased for business or promotional use or for special sales. For information, please write to: Special Markets Department, Random House, Inc., 1540 Broadway, New York, NY 10036.

BROADWAY BOOKS and its logo, a letter B bisected on the diagonal, are trademarks of Broadway Books, a division of Random House, Inc.

Visit our Web site at www.broadwaybooks.com

First Broadway Books trade paperback edition published 2000.

IMPORTANT NOTE: The reader should bear in mind that this book is not intended to take the place of medical advice from a trained medical professional. Readers are advised to consult a physician or other qualified health professional regarding treatment of all their health problems. This book was written to provide selected information to the public concerning conventional and alternative medical treatments. Research in this field is ongoing and subject to interpretation. Neither the publisher nor the author takes responsibility for any possible consequences from any treatment, action, or use of herbs, medicine, or other substance by any person reading or following the information in this book.

Sodium, Potassium, Calcium Chart used courtesy of Joseph E. Pizzorno, Jr., N.D., Bastyr University

Designed by Donna Sinisgalli

Sullivan, Andrea D.
A path to healing: a guide to wellness for body, mind, and soul/
Andrea D. Sullivan.—1st ed.
p. cm.
Includes index.
1. Naturopathy.   2. Alternative medicine.   3. Afro-Americans—
Health and hygiene.   I. Title.
RZ440.S84   1998
615.5'35—dc21   97-47063
                              CIP

ISBN 0-385-48577-8
Copyright © 1998 by Andrea D. Sullivan
All Rights Reserved
Printed in the United States of America

10   9   8   7   6   5   4   3

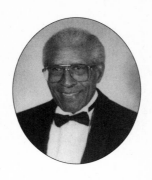

THIS BOOK IS DEDICATED

to the memories of my father,

Walter Theodis Sullivan, Sr.,

and to my great-grandmother,

"Mama T," Mrs. Mary S. Tribbitt

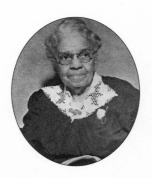

The Lord hath created medicines out of the earth;
and he that is wise will not abhor them.

—Ecclesiasticus 38:4

Medicus curat, natura sanat—*Medicine treats, but nature heals.*

—Pare

I Am Grateful

"Mama T," Mrs. Mary S. Tribbitt, my great-grandmother, was known for her missionary work in Philadelphia, specifically fund-raising to establish the first home for unwed mothers, which opened in 1925. Mama T believed that "what we call a bad girl is only a good girl who has made a mistake. It's then she needs a friend." She was spirited and fearless, commanding the attention of minds and the goodness of hearts. She's one of several in my family who planted seeds of passion, determination, strength, and discipline along my path to healing.

I could not have walked this path but for the dignity and grace extended to me through Spirit in the form of my parents, Mary Lucretia and Walter Theodis, and their loving presence, guidance, and support throughout my life; for the strength and sacrifice of their parents, Ellen and John, and Verda and William; and their parents . . . "Mama T" . . .

As my path has lead me into the writing of this book, I have continued to be blessed by all of my family, and many friends who care. I cannot name you all, but you know who you are. Thank you. But to Walter and Sean, I say thank you for loving me, serenading me with "Stomp," and choosing to be a part of my family. And to my dear friends Vera Smith and Ellen Collins I say thank you for the years of caring and support, for always being there, and allowing me to be who I am.

And I extend my gratitude to those who have walked closely with me on this part of my journey:

Michael Evanson, my forever friend, for guiding me to Brooklyn to meet Dr. James D'Adamo, laughing with me when crying was an option, and loving me no matter what;

Dr. James D'Adamo, my friend, colleague, and mentor, for being remarkably accurate about my purpose in life;

All of my patients, for their trust and faith in natural medicine;

Gail Ross, my attorney, who asked me to write an "herbal book," but believed in my ideas to create something bigger;

Howard Yoon, my editor, whose quiet strength, direction, and computer literacy made many moments easier;

Gaynell Catherine, my researcher, for having all of the answers, anytime, night or day;

Karen Harris, my assistant, who spent endless hours in conversations about, and in manuscript preparation of, Part I of "the book";

Marilyn Milloy and Joseph Windham, my patients, for assisting me with "Naturopathy: The Roots";

Janet Hill, Senior Editor at Doubleday, whose wisdom and vision allowed me to keep my focus, and whose sense of humor made the time spent on this project much more fun.

Heart and Soul,
Andrea Sullivan

Contents

Introduction

At age twenty-nine I thought I was living the American dream. I had a Ph.D. in sociology, a high-level job in the Department of Housing and Urban Development, and, as if that were not enough, the antique Mercedes-Benz I had always wanted. Yet one day in 1978, as I was leaning against the doorframe of my HUD office, I realized that something in my life was very wrong.

That was the day I watched Milton Street, an activist for homeless people, carefully assist an elderly woman off one of the many buses parked near the HUD building. The scene had given me a glimpse of a different reality. Yes, I was a special assistant to the Secretary of HUD, responsible for urban policy and crime prevention, and yes, I had all the trinkets that come with success. But I felt empty and ill at ease. My colleagues and I had been instructed to offer Street false promises to help the homeless in order to avoid a protest in front of the HUD building.

The harsh reality of my situation became clearer when I told the Secretary I didn't agree with the plan to deceive these homeless people and their advocates. She became upset and threatened to terminate my employment for insubordination. In that moment I became aware of being dispensable. I understood that my life could be different with the stroke of a pen, that my success at HUD could end without completing my life goal of doing something meaningful for people. But had I spent all those years in school to participate in a system that trades compassion for deception?

The experience of that day had a profound effect on me. I had already questioned my role and my effectiveness in the HUD bureaucracy. I was exhausted from the long hours I spent pursuing meaningless answers to problems that begged substantive solutions. I asked myself what kind of success I had attained and at what cost. I was dis-*eased*.

Not sick in the traditional sense of the word: there was no fever, there were no diseases in any organs. But I had no energy. I was worn out, thirty pounds overweight, and though I was well past my adolescent years, my face was covered with acne. I was also ill at ease spiritually and emotionally. I didn't feel *whole.*

How could I help create success in the world? One thing—perhaps the only thing—I was sure of was that I wanted to make a positive difference in the lives of the people on this planet. How could I help others, I asked myself, if I was not well?

I knew I needed help from a health professional but, like many people, I was wary of turning to the world of conventional medicine. A lot of people, black people in particular, mistrust the health care system; we fear that the legacy that has deprived us of equal treatment in so many other arenas also exists in hospitals and doctors' offices. I knew that, while I needed physical healing, I also needed something more, something I was not likely to get from the doctors I had gone to before. So began a journey that would change my life.

A good friend referred me to James D'Adamo, N.D., who practiced naturopathic medicine. Naturopathic doctors use natural remedies to fight illness and prescribe lifestyle changes to prevent disease. Naturopaths treat *people,* not diseases. They believe that the body has an innate ability to heal itself if given proper support and nutrients. The terms "holistic doctors" and "holistic health" have their origin in naturopathic medicine, or nature cure. Holistic medicine has come to mean anything from preventive medicine, which focuses on early detection through screening, Pap smears, and the use of some vitamins and drugs, to naturopathy, which emphasizes *primary prevention*—that is, prevention *before* the occurrence of disease and treatment with relatively nontoxic agents such as vitamins, minerals, herbs, and foods that support physiologic function. Because the total organism is involved in healing, the most effective approach, like naturopathy, considers and treats the whole person. A naturopath pays careful attention to an individual's life conditions and one's susceptibility to disease.

Naturopaths work with patients to remedy the causes, not just the outward signs, of their illnesses. My doctor spent a long time talking to me in an effort to find out why I wasn't well. Through my sessions with him, I learned that much of my "disease" had to do with the experiences I had endured as an African-American. He learned that, despite good grades, my high school counselor had told me that I should become a maid. He learned of the shame and humiliation I felt when my white friends in high school hid me in their basements when their parents came home. He learned that I, like many African-Americans, believed I was invisible to most of society.

I began my path toward wellness through natural remedies. Within six months I was physically and emotionally better. I felt more in control of my life, and I wondered how the herbs and foods and homeopathic remedies were working. Why did I feel so different?

During my first visit with Dr. D'Adamo, he had suggested that I become a naturopath. "Just give me some bat feathers and whatever else you have and I'll be on my way back to D.C.," I quickly answered. I had a career, I told him, and I wasn't interested in yet another degree. I thought of his words every day as my acne faded and my body took on a new, healthier shape. Increasingly frustrated with my lack of authority at work, I was compelled by the feeling of empowerment that resulted from my new, naturopathic lifestyle. By becoming a naturopath, I realized, I could provide a truly valuable service to others, sharing with them this life-changing experience.

After two years at Howard University in Washington, where I fulfilled the prerequisites, I sold all the vestiges of material success, including my prized Benz, and moved to Seattle to study naturopathy at Bastyr University, one of the world's preeminent educational centers of natural healing. The first two years were grueling: thirty hours of class time in biochemistry, physiology, immunology, and anatomy each week, in addition to introductory courses on naturopathy.

I experienced additional stress by being the only African-American in the school. I felt responsible to represent all blacks. I had no friends or family in Seattle and saw very few black people. (Seattle's population was about 8 percent black.) Exhausted and lonely, I came home between my second and third year of school. I was again broken, but this time I had a mission, something to strive for.

I had come home for nurturing, support, and rest. Most of all, I needed to nurture myself—to focus on my spirit and inner feelings to create a sense of wholeness. I participated in personal growth seminars and read all the self-help and spiritual books I could find.

Then, while I was still away from school, I took a spiritual pilgrimage with a group of friends of all ethnicities, to Jerusalem, Egypt, and

Assisi. I spent seven weeks chanting inside the top of the great pyramid, looking into the eyes of Egyptians while they shared their meager possessions with me; walking the path of Jesus Christ from Pilate's judgment hall to the place of crucifixion; meditating at the Mount of Olives and in the Garden of Gethsemane; living on a kibbutz in Israel and being in awe of and humbled by the life of St. Francis of Assisi. This pilgrimage helped me realize who I really was.

More importantly, I realized God is love. God is in everything and everyone. I would never be alone again. I needed only to reach out and share because I was a part of everything too. I had a renewed vision of how I wanted to help others. By the time I returned to school I was physically and spiritually rejuvenated, and full of gratitude for finally understanding why we are here on this planet and my role in this world.

My next two years at Bastyr included courses that were at the heart of naturopathic medicine, such as counseling, nutrition, herbal and homeopathic medicine, and acupuncture. Each course was more exciting than the last. During my clinical work, seeing a patient's health improve was one of the most fulfilling experiences in my life. I had found my home in this gentle healing art.

As the years pass since my graduation in 1986, I have become more aware of my own healing process and how each step in the journey toward my degree was full of necessary experiences. I am grateful. Today I have a busy homeopathic and naturopathic practice with a three-month waiting list. I am a diplomate of the Homeopathic Academy of Naturopathic Physicians, a founding member of the American Association of Naturopathic Physicians, and a member of both the National Center for Homeopathy and the International Foundation for Homeopathy. I have appeared on many television and radio shows and speak regularly to national professional organizations, church and civic groups around Washington, D.C., where I live and work.

One of my reasons for writing this book is that, just as conventional medicine has been too willing to overlook the needs of African-American people, so has naturopathy. There is a dearth of information on this subject that includes African-American patients, and too little has been written by African-American professionals about it. As African-Americans' contributions have been excluded from American history books, so has the African-Americans' involvement been excluded from the texts on natural and herbal medicine. Not only can naturopathy compensate in some part for the inadequate conventional health care people of color and poor people sometimes face, it can correct some of the unhealthy lifestyles and beliefs that are at the root of many diseases common to all Americans.

This book is not to judge, justify, or minimize the behaviors or experiences that anyone or any group of people has had. It is to give me an opportunity to share with you information I have learned about people and healing that I hope will enable you to expand your consciousness and create healing. I hope to assist people in healing themselves through naturopathic techniques they can perform at home. I will teach readers about the natural remedies, homeopathy, proper nutrition, personal-growth techniques, and stress-reduction techniques that changed my life. But before I do so, I will address the uniqueness of the history of this country that shaped the behavior of our ancestors. It is that behavior that affects our well-being and creates dis-ease.

AN AMERICAN EXPERIENCE

In 1705, under Virginia law, a master who killed a slave while disciplining him was not charged with a crime. The law stated that the master ". . . shall be free and acquit of all punishment and accusation for the same, as if such accident had never happened." What is the result of such a heinous law? What effect does this have on all people governed by this law? Arguments in favor of the slave Sommersett, in the Sommersett v. Stuart case of 1771, provide us with an answer. One of the attorneys for Sommersett, Mr. Francis Hargrave, said the following (the italics for emphasis are mine):

> Slavery *corrupts the morals* of the master, by freeing him from those restraints with respect to his slave, so necessary for *control of the human passions*, so beneficial in promoting the practice and *confirming the habit of virtue*—it is dangerous to the master, because his oppression excites implacable resentment and hatred in the slave. . . . To the slave it communicates all the afflictions of life . . . and it depresses the excellence of his nature. . . . It is dangerous to the state, by its corruption of those citizens on whom its prosperity depends; and by admitting within it a

multitude of persons, who being excluded from the common benefits of the constitution are interested in scheming its destruction. Hence it is, that slavery, in whatever light we view it, may be deemed a most pernicious institution; immediately so, to the unhappy person who suffers under it; finally so, to the master who triumphs in it, and to the state which allows it.

This quote is key to any explanation of the beginning of dis-ease in this country. Slavery corrupted the master's principles with respect to his behavior, and allowed for freedom of his emotion, lust, and desire. There was no constraint on conduct; right and wrong had no meaning. What must it do to the psyche of a person to be able to treat another without regard for that person's life? What happened to the psyche of the master and the slave? When behavior has no boundaries or limits, discipline and compassion are lost. This behavior was visited upon not only the slaves but also families, all families. The master could not confine his lawless passions to the slave; thus, the master's wife and children were familiar with abuse as well.

And whether by imitation or direct learning, the offspring of the masters were also taught the same corruption of morals and lack of control. Similarly, the slave learned, and taught his descendants, what was learned from the master—how to be a slave, replete with a very different self-esteem and sense of identity.

Slavery was an *American* experience, not only a black American experience—a process of dehumanization, humiliation, deprivation, and thwarted ambition for black Africans, and behaviors founded upon unbridled passions and fear for European-Americans. Its consequences linger. Specifically, for some African-American men, a lack of responsibility and a sense of powerlessness. For most African-American women, a legacy of surviving and keeping families together at *all* costs. For European-American women, a dependency and sense of inadequacy because her value and role in life were minimized. For European-American men, a false sense of power and superiority that is fueled by the subordination of others.

Through the generations we have seen the results of the moral depravity of slavery. The behavior of the people of this country has been, and continues to be, shaped by this institution, and its legacy of fear and violence continues to plague our society. Racism is one of the most destructive and violent sources of sickness in America. All of us are victims of the disease of racism. Today, blacks and whites alike experience the same feelings of alienation, insecurity, fear, despair, and self-deprecation that resulted from an institution based on hatred.

Day after day I hear the accounts of my patients' lives. Without looking at them, in some instances, I could not determine their ethnicity. There is a common theme to many of the stories—fear, isolation, worthlessness, anxiety, and abuse (drugs, alcohol, sexual, physical). Each person—black or white—could tell the other person's story. It seems pain has no preference regarding where it resides. The effect of abuse and neglect, whether it is directed toward a people for hundreds of years or toward a single person for eighteen years, is damaging.

That is why this book is not simply prescriptive; it is not only for the purpose of teaching you how to use herbs for a particular condition. But rather it is to emphasize that healing has to come from deep within us, where dis-ease begins. Healing has to happen at the core of ourselves where the insults, shame, hurt feelings, and anger of the past reside. Health requires replacing this core with soundness and wholeness. Freedom from the darkness—in mood, word, and deed—and freedom from the separation in our hearts is what I am seeking for us all.

Consider Catherine, a middle-aged black woman who came to my practice suffering from weight loss and fatigue. She was well educated, articulate, and easy to get along with.

As I do with all my patients on their initial visits, I spent an hour and a half talking with Catherine. Slowly, as she responded to my questions about her life, a devastating story emerged. She had been working in a government agency for nearly twenty years. Twice in the past five years she had been passed over for promotion. In both cases, Catherine had trained the individuals who got the promotion and in both cases the individuals were white. When Catherine was recently turned down for a third promotion, this time to a white male with less education and less than half her work experience, Catherine felt utterly defeated and depressed. Her body had finally succumbed to the stress that this situation had caused her; she became exhausted and lost her appetite.

Women of all ethnicities suffer from job discrimination, as it was but one of the motivating factors of the women's movement. And many of the participants in the civil rights movement were Caucasian Americans who experienced racism and discrimination as abominable. Martha, a Caucasian patient, said to me once, "I have strong feelings about racism. What the European culture has done and continues to do to people of color is shameful. And what white men have done to all of us in this country is obscene." Martha's story is one of loneliness and abuse. Her dis-ease manifested itself in high cholesterol, high blood pressure, and about fifty extra and unwanted pounds. Martha came from a family in which she felt "manipulated, lied to, and misrepresented." Her mother had recently died. She wept as she told me, "All of my life my mother told me that my father did not care for me and that is why he never came to see me. It was not until I was in my thirties that I found out that my mother prevented my father from seeing me." Her mother was manic depressive and an "over-the-counter drug addict," and her father was alcoholic. Martha's home life was in constant turmoil. It was up to Martha to maintain order in the home and care for her younger brother and sister. "I was the mother. My mother told me her problems and cared little about my life. When she was depressed, she'd just lay around and holler at me to do this and that." Martha felt isolated and unloved much of the time, and at age seventeen she left home. She married at a young age to a man who was also an alcoholic and living with someone else part time. Martha discovered the infidelity by chance. He was verbally abusive and very disrespectful. "I was very dependent on him. I only spoke when he allowed me to speak." After their separation he did not pay child support for any of their three children. Martha was devastated by her life's experiences and was seeking my assistance to lower her blood pressure and reduce her weight, anxiety, and depression.

If Martha feels isolated, and poor eating habits put her at risk for obesity and the diseases that come with it, she cannot do the work necessary to guide her children or herself on the path to healing. She cannot keep her sons and daughters from the dangers of alcohol and drugs.

If the stresses Catherine endures as an African-American in the workplace immobilize her, or if she responds to those stresses with unhealthy diet or negative behavior, rather than coping with them in a positive way, she will not be effective in challenging the system that unfairly denied her a job promotion. Her feelings of worthlessness will be reinforced, and the cycle will continue.

Isolation, worthlessness, and discrimination are not limited by color but are American experiences. There is much work yet to be done, and poor health will hamper the effort.

A TIME FOR NEW CHOICES

What do my own experiences as an African-American and my practice in naturopathic healing have to do with Martha's and Catherine's stories? To Catherine, losing the promotion had been "a slap in the face," in her words; calling into question her self-worth and self-esteem. To Martha, having a drug-addicted mother and alcoholic father created a sense of rejection, mistrust, and uncertainty, often feeling what she believed or experienced did not matter to anyone in her family. As a naturopathic physician, I believe the experiences of these women represented one of the reasons for their illness and these experiences are directly related to the institution of slavery and the history of this country. Catherine's feelings of worthlessness made her sick. Repeated discrimination based on color precipitated Catherine's feelings of dis-ease. Martha's feelings of isolation and rejection made her sick. Her mother's manic depression was a result of the powerlessness and abuse she suffered at the hands of her parents. Her father's alcoholism was a result of his need to escape the pain of his childhood: having had a critical and abusive father. The feelings of these women made them engage in unhealthy behaviors, such as eating a poor diet or having negative thoughts. The effects of these stressors are debilitating. I see this in my practice among my patients who have endured experiences such as Martha's and Catherine's.

As we approach the twenty-first century, we all need to take responsibility for healing ourselves. Americans cannot afford to do nothing and hope that a system whose origins were based on hatred and profoundly devoid of feeling and morality, a system that never intended for part of its citizenry to be included in the system, will create a meaningful difference for all of us today.

We cannot depend on "society" to make choices for us. We are society. We need to create physical, emotional, mental, and spiritual wellness for ourselves through techniques I will describe. Out of that wellness will come a myriad of opportunities that will not materialize if we are ill or feeling so worthless that we do not want to get out of bed in the morning, much less be able to meet life's challenges.

We do not always take sufficient advantage of our power of choice. If we continue to do what we have always done, we will continue to get what we have always gotten. Many still choose to let stress overwhelm their bodies and encourage unhealthy behavior. The violence in our society is a direct result of our sense of isolation, disregard for ourselves, and disrespect for the lives of others, many of the ingredients that fueled the institution of slavery. Homicide, for example, is among the leading causes of death for young black males in America. In this age of violence among all youths, Americans need to be aware that research has shown a correlation between poor diet and juvenile delinquency. When my patients tell me they cannot afford to buy their groceries at a health food store, I tell them they cannot afford not to. As one of my elderly patients told me, you can pay the grocer or you can pay the doctor. We must make different choices.

We need to choose health care providers who will see us as whole beings and who will consider all the experiences that have contributed to our diseases. We need to seek the counsel of physicians who will listen to us, hear what we are saying, and provide appropriate remedies. We need to heed the advice of physicians who will help us heal ourselves.

WHY NATUROPATHY?

Why naturopathy? Because for centuries naturopathy—even though it wasn't called that at the time—cured ills when no other medical care was available. As you will read in Chapter Two, "Naturopathy: The Roots," Americans have a rich history of knowledge about herbs and other natural remedies that have healed through the generations. While it is not widely known, for years Africans were "doctors" to their masters and their masters' children, and their treatments were found in nature, similar to those used in Africa. Today, the benefits of many such remedies are well documented. In fact, many of the drugs used in conventional medicine come from plants, for example foxglove or digitalis, that are used to treat heart conditions.

Why naturopathy? Because too many Americans still have limited access to conventional health care, and understanding preventive health care is vital. Because conventional drugs, which often contain synthetic elements or are given in high doses, do more harm than good to some people. Because in some situations the unintended (side) effects of conventional drugs can be devastating. Because too often conventional physicians prefer to focus on artificially prolonging life through invasive, high-tech treatments rather than avoiding disease and suffering through healthy lifestyles and gentle but effective natural remedies.

We should consider naturopathy because the diseases that run rampant in America did not develop overnight, in a vacuum, and the healing measures must reflect that. Naturopathy recognizes that the challenges people face can have profound effects on their bodies' defenses.

More and more often I see children who are disruptive and violent or who have poor concentration. Black or white, rich or poor, they have a need to belong; they tell me they feel unloved and alone, as their lives have already been challenging. Their self-esteem has been molded by the absentee father or the workaholic father (also absentee), and a mother who is stressed out and feeling inadequate. This is not the way it was when I was a child. We had gangs of friends back then, but the gangs did not have guns. We had disagreements with our peers over a jacket or a pair of shoes, but we asked our teachers to settle our arguments. We did not kill the person with whom we disagreed. But today, increasing numbers of children engage in manic, violent behavior. Many children with manic behavior who are treated by conventional physicians are put on drugs that often make them sluggish and unproductive, unable to participate fully in life. In naturopathic medicine there are gentler alternatives for treating some disruptive and violent behavior. It is worth noting again that the relationship between diet and juvenile delinquency is well documented. Making changes in what we eat can oftentimes change our behavior. And homeopathic treatment has allowed many children to discontinue Ritalin, the drug prescribed for children diagnosed with Attention Deficit Disorder.

While it is also true that many people choose only naturopathy for treatment just as people choose only conventional medicine, these forms of medicine can and do complement each other. Naturopathic medicine is *complementary* medicine, not simply "alternative" medicine, and can be used along with conventional medicine for treatment of any condition; conventional drugs do not always have to be the first line of defense. The keepers of mainstream medicine would lead us to believe that naturopathy is an alternative form of medicine and that the patient must choose one or the other. You do not have to choose. You will see in the second part of this book that I use homeopathy, herbs, and nutrition for patients who are taking all types of drugs, from chemotherapy for cancer to hydrochlorothiazide for high blood pressure. Herbs, foods, and homeopathy are natural. They do not in any way interfere with synthetic drugs, but rather complement the process of healing that the body is attempting, despite the suppression and devastation that steroids and chemotherapy, for example, may cause. Whatever choices you make about your health, it is *your* choice and *your* responsibility. Choose wisely.

Heal Your Neighbor, Heal Yourself

The Dalai Lama said, "In today's highly interdependent world, individuals and nations can no longer resolve many of their problems by themselves. We need one another. We must therefore develop a sense of universal responsibility. . . . It is our collective and individual responsibility to protect and nurture the global family, to support its weaker members and to preserve and tend to the environment in which we all live."

Virtually all the world's spiritual writings teach that *we are one people and one race—the human race*. Sogyal Rinpoche, in *The Tibetan Book of Living and Dying*, says: "True spirituality also is to be aware that if we are interdependent with everything and everyone else, even our smallest, least significant thought, word, and action have real consequences throughout the universe. . . . Everything is inextricably interrelated: We come to realize we are responsible for everything we do, say, or think, responsible in fact for ourselves, everyone and everything else, and the entire universe." In *A Path to Healing*, I will share with you my understanding of how we are all connected and how important it is to use that understanding as an antidote to the dis-ease that discrimination and isolation create.

The healing I teach in this book is directed to all Americans and applies to all people, regardless of color. But because of my heritage and the disproportionate amount of illness in blacks, I feel a responsibility to highlight certain issues throughout the book that are specific to that community, issues that I hope will educate and promote a greater understanding between all ethnic groups. Black people suffer deeply from denial that we are part of the human race. This denial created a dis-ease of the soul that extends into the mental, emotional, and physical bodies of each of us. It is a denial of our interconnectedness. When one of us is harmed, we are all affected. Dr. King once said:

> We realize that injustice anywhere is a threat to justice everywhere. Our destiny is bound up with the destiny of America—we built it for two centuries without wages. . . . We built our homes and homes for our masters and suffered injustice and humiliation. We feel that we are all the conscience of America. We are its troubled soul. We must learn to live together as brothers or perish together as fools.

We identify ourselves in terms of individuals, groups, and affiliations. Too often, because of the history of this country, people are seen in terms of ethnicity, religious or sexual orientation, rather than as individuals. We ignore the essence and focus on the shell. Ethnicities, whether white, black, yellow, or red, more often than not have stereotypes attached to them, and those stereotypes interfere with our ability to see our oneness. We do not see ourselves as a community of God's people, of God's children, of sisters and brothers. But rather we see one another as the enemy. Hatred is the enemy. Hatred is crippling and weakening this country. Hatred can make you sick. Hatred is bred from ignorance—the ignorance of not knowing ourselves and each other. African-Americans are easily identifiable, and more stereotypes are based on ethnicity than on any other identity. In defense, or because of some discomfort they feel, often I hear people say, "I don't see color when I look at you." I say that is unfortunate. I want you to recognize I am African-American and respect, appreciate, and celebrate that fact as I would celebrate you, and be eager to know you, your history, challenges, and victories.

So, in addition to poor dietary habits and negative thinking, another habit that Americans must break is the separation of the "races." Maya Angelou, in her book, *Wouldn't Take Nothing for My Journey Now*, tells us that Americans need to be aware of and experience other countries and cultures so that we can see our human likeness even though we may have different philosophies and speak different languages. She says: "Perhaps travel cannot prevent bigotry, but by demonstrating that all peoples cry, laugh, eat, worry, and die, it can introduce the idea that if we try to understand each other we may even become friends."

It is time that we understand clearly and embrace the goodness and wealth that can be gleaned from respecting and participating in the diversity of this country, alive in all people. Unless we *all* clean up our act we will always be poor in spirit, begging, and unhappy. We will have addictions, crime, and dis-ease. Do not fool yourself, we are *all* affected when babies are born to drug-addicted mothers, when children kill, and when people live on the grates of our cities. No one is free from thought, or worry, whether it is conscious or unconscious.

We will not achieve healing by blaming and despising others for their actions; we will achieve it by empowering ourselves. The issue is not whether black people can forgive white people for what they have done in the past; rather, people who have engaged in discrimination and racism, whether black or white, must forgive themselves so that they too can heal this wound. When we heal ourselves, we heal our neighbors, and when we heal our neighbors, we help to heal the ailing body of humankind.

Where does the healing begin? Healing begins inside each of us. It begins with knowing that we deserve a healthy, prosperous life full of grace. It may be a slow and difficult process, but we must begin somewhere. "If you can't fly, run. If you can't run, walk. If you can't walk, crawl. But by all means keep moving," Dr. King once said.

Each of us can take responsibility for our own wellness not only through nutrition, stress reduction, and natural therapies, but also by thinking healthier thoughts, speaking kinder words, and participating in greater acts of service. The atrocities left in the wake of the institution of slavery have left an indelible stain on the psyches of Americans both black and white, but nonetheless slavery is a part of our heritage. Our birthright, however, as children of God is abundance and joy, not pain and suffering. Because we have been taught to think otherwise, we must break old habits and form new ones that are rich in the goodness of life.

This book will not right all social wrongs or miraculously reverse all disease. It will not end racism or discrimination. But it will provide a foundation for a journey on the path to healing. The information here will fortify you so that you can respond to life with greater purpose and intention. Its suggestions will empower you. It is a journey that I too have made, and my prayers will be with you as you embark on yours. I wish you Godspeed and good health.

PART ONE

REFLECTIONS
ON HEALTH

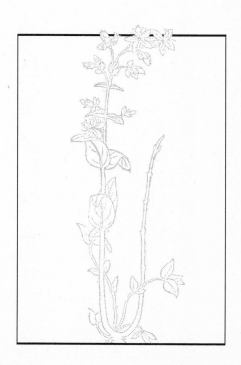

1

WHAT IS HEALTH?
A NATUROPATHIC PERSPECTIVE

"I have been joyful and my health is good. Now I think right, exercise, and eat right. When you laugh a lot you feel energized."

—*A Patient*

When I ask my patients how they are the answer is usually "Fine." I continue by asking, "What does 'fine' mean?" Then the answer becomes, "I'm okay." When I ask for more clarification many will say, "I don't have any physical ailments but I'm not doing that good. I just don't feel *well.*" Many people you know will respond the same way. We are used to feeling unwell, as if that were healthy. The truth is many people don't know what it is like to wake up feeling well rested (and not needing coffee), focused, and optimistic with a sense of peace.

Health is a process, a continuum from wellness (optimal health) to illness to death. Many people believe wellness is simply an absence of symptoms. But health is more than just a physical condition. It is to be in harmony with oneself, one's environment, and one's God. It means being flexible with and accepting of ourselves and others. It involves ways in which we think about and treat ourselves and others. To be well is to have a consciousness of loving for yourself and others. It is to know that you are worthy of having wealth in the form of good health, loving relationships, and prosperity. Being well means recognizing that you are provided for because you are God's child. Good health is trusting the process of life, knowing that everything is perfect even when we don't like it. Good health is physical and psychological vitality, a passion and enthusiasm that lead to an overall sense of wellness and gratitude for the blessings in life. No matter how negative things may appear, there is gratitude for what is good about life. Usually accompanied by feelings of joy, happiness, and love, good health is absence of dis-ease (a lack of ease or feeling of being ill at ease which is not always or necessarily the same as *disease*), as well as absence of symptoms. When we are truly well, a few physical symptoms are not enough to make us feel unhealthy or ill. Good health is a right. You are entitled to it.

Health is freedom from spiritual, mental, emotional, and physical limitations. Spiritual and mental freedom is the ability to express oneself creatively without egocentrism and to think clearly with compassion and will. Emotionally healthy people are free to experience a wide range of feelings: grief, anger, anxiety. They are able to feel these emotions and yet be detached from them, maintaining an underlying sense of inner peace and balance. Not dwelling on any one emotion, they leave themselves open to the next moment; they experience the fullness of life.

Creating good health is not the responsibility of the doctor or pharmaceutical companies as conventional medicine has led us to believe. Good health is our responsibility. Because of the stress of lifestyles, foods, and negative thoughts, most of us are operating below zero on a health scale of one to ten. My job is to assist people in getting back up to "one" using homeopathy, nutrition, and herbs so that they can then support themselves through the rest of the process. We are in a partnership that involves changing their lifestyles; the patient does the work as well as the healing, I am simply the facilitator. This attitude about wellness comes from our basic naturopathic beliefs, based on principles of vitalism.

ALLOPATHIC VS. NATUROPATHIC PHILOSOPHY

In allopathic or traditional medicine, symptoms of disease are thought to be a result of a physiologic reaction to bacteria or viruses; symptoms are considered destructive and must be controlled or eliminated so that order can be restored. When the symptoms disappear, it is assumed that the disease has been eradicated or at least controlled.

When drugs are given they work against the body's attempt to heal itself. There certainly are times when bacteria must be destroyed rapidly and mechanical intervention—or surgery—is necessary. However, the body needs to be supported in its effort to increase resistance and decrease susceptibility. Drugs relieve symptoms but do not stimulate or encourage healing. Quite the contrary: continuous intervention leads to suppression of the body's natural ability to heal and can produce undesirable effects. One example is the rampant use of prophylactic antibiotics for children with ear infections. These children show up regularly in my practice with diarrhea and nausea because the normal bacterial flora of the body, *Lactobacillus acidophilus,* has been eliminated by the antibiotic and, as a result, yeast is allowed to flourish in the intestines. Unfortunately, for many of these kids the earaches still occur, which leads to further use of antibiotics. The cycle thus continues.

Naturopathic medicine (which is *complementary,* not alternative, medicine) is based on the philosophy of vitalism. Vitalism maintains that life is more than a complex series of chemical and physical reactions. It relies on a belief that there is a soul, that which makes us breathe, that coordinates and organizes these reactions. This force, or *vitalism,* allows an organism to develop, reproduce, and repair itself.

Naturopaths believe that the symptoms of a disease are not solely the result of bacteria or a virus, but the body's inherent response to it. Symptoms are indicators of the body's attempt to eradicate this harmful agent. They reflect the innate intelligence of an organism to maintain wellness. Our bodies strive to maintain homeostasis (the maintenance of stability and constancy while adapting to changes, such as extreme temperatures). Those of us in natural or complementary medicine appreciate symptoms because they are signs that the body is creating resistance to the bacteria. In treating a sick patient, we try to stimulate the body's ability to respond to the offending agent and repair itself.

This is not to say that naturopathy does not at times support the use of drugs in some situations. But the use of natural therapies means there is little suppression of the immune system and there are few unintended effects. Within the scope of naturopathy, the body's healing power is never thwarted. Naturopathic remedies seek to strengthen and support the body's innate healing power.

Differing Perspectives of Health

Because of underlying differences in their philosophies, allopaths and naturopaths (including homeopaths) view health from different perspectives. Allopaths have a philosophy of illness. They base their understanding of sickness on the germ theory. They believe bacteria or viruses cause disease and that symptoms are the disease itself. It is not until the symptoms localize to a specific organ that allopaths classify and diagnose the disease. They usually treat the disease with drugs or surgery, and measure the success of the treatment when the symptoms go away. Oftentimes success is achieved by any means necessary, no matter how dangerous the drug.

Naturopathy, on the other hand, focuses on health or wellness. I would determine your wellness through conversation, by noting your emotional, spiritual, and physical well-being, and by assessing risk factors such as social and emotional stress and nutritional deficiencies. As a classical homeopathic physician I want to know the stresses in your life, issues and challenges you have had to overcome and what effect you believe those challenges had on your body, mind, and emotions. I want to know your fears, sleep patterns, and food cravings as well. For example, I may ask you why you believe you have this condition. What was occurring in your life at the time of or five years before the onset of the disease? What makes you angry or sad and what is your behavior when you are angry or sad? Or are you impatient or irritable? Because we know that a change in one part of the body creates change in another, we must study the whole organism.

Symptoms signal a disturbance in the body. A symptom is not a disease or the cause of a disease, but a way for the body to defend itself and keep itself well. It is the best reaction that your body can make when it comes in contact with a bacterium or virus or any stress. Fever, for example, is a symptom that all of us are familiar with. It is an important defense mechanism which stimulates the body's white blood cells and secretions of interferon, both of which help fight infection. By getting rid of the fever, I would suppress the body's natural defenses. And more importantly, I would not have addressed the original cause of the disturbance.

Rather than controlling the disease or wiping out the symptom, naturopaths work to support and strengthen the body's natural healing mechanisms in order to decrease susceptibility. Naturopaths refer to susceptibility as the organism's degree of strength against offending agents. It is determined by levels of mental, emotional, and physical stress.

LIFESTYLE CHANGES

Naturopathic medicine seeks to normalize bodily functions, restore a state of wellness, and prevent disease. The philosophy of *vis medicatrix naturae,* the healing power of nature, is fundamental to naturopathic medicine. Using everything that nature provides, I cooperate and support the body's innate ability to heal itself. As a naturopath I avoid the use of drugs and procedures that interrupt normal function and have unintended negative (side) effects. I use nontoxic therapies based on physiologic principles to treat the whole individual, not just the disease or condition, because the whole person is involved in the healing process. My concern is with the cause, treatment, and prevention of disease.

Naturopathic doctors teach patients to make lifestyle changes that focus on proper nutrition, elimination of drugs and alcohol, stress reduction, exercise, rest, and recreation. As you will read in subsequent chapters, besides a homeopathic remedy, my patients are given strategies for taking responsibility for their health, such as dietary recommendations, stress reduction techniques, and herbal and vitamin prescriptions for specific diseases. I am a primary care physician working in concert with patients to establish good health habits.

Naturopathic philosophy believes that whatever is going on inside and outside your body can minimize or maximize health. Most disease begins because of violation of these laws. The laws include eating natural unprocessed foods, getting adequate rest and exercise, having a positive attitude, living a moderately paced lifestyle, and avoiding polluted environments. Benedict Lust, who brought naturopathy to the United States in 1902, wrote in the *Naturopathic and Herald of Health* (1902):

> We plead for the renunciation of poisons from the coffee, white flour, glucose (sugar), lard and like venom of the American table to patent medicines, tobacco, liquor and other inevitable

recourse of perverted appetite. We long for a time when an eight-hour day may enable every worker to stop existing long enough to live; when the spirit of universal brotherhood shall animate business and society and the church . . . when people may stop doing and thinking and being for others and be for themselves. . . .

The scope of naturopathy is broad because we treat people, not diseases. Every phase of life is important to the naturopath. We treat everyone from the infant to the elderly, using therapies such as homeopathy, nutrition, botanicals (herbs), acupuncture, hydrotherapy, exercise, manipulation, and massage. Our specialties then are in these treatments that we use and not in organ systems such as the heart, cardiology, the joints, or rheumatology as in conventional medicine.

As Lust said in 1902:

In a word, Naturopathy stands for the reconciling, harmonizing and unifying of nature, humanity and God. Fundamentally therapeutic because men need healing; elementally educational because men need teaching; ultimately inspirational because men need empowering, it encompasses the realm of human progress and destiny. . . .

Many Americans are changing their lifestyles to what Lust advised. Over the last several decades we have seen a resurgence of naturopathic medicine. I say resurgence because it is not new.

2

NATUROPATHY:
THE ROOTS

Colored folks was brought up on these old home remedies. Like I tell
you 'bout this fever grass-hump. You know when folks in the
community—lots of 'em would make that fever grass the same day or
night and give it to 'em. You know we stayed up too, with the chillun;
didn't have no doctors. These old home remedies; that's all I ever took.
Right now, you know, I ain't never been to a doctor.
                    —Mildred Graves, 84, Macon County, Alabama

It happens all the time in my practice: African-American patients, when
pondering my prescription for wellness through herbs, recount how a
grandmother or aunt or great-uncle used herbal remedies. For precisely
what condition of the body or spirit, or with what herbs exactly, patients
usually don't know or can't remember. But they remember relatives
taking these natural remedies as their primary form of medicine.

This doesn't surprise me. For years I was vaguely aware of a certain
"yellowbush" my grandmother told me her mother boiled and dispensed to her children for colds and influenza. But I never knew the
name of this magical shrub. Was it chamomile, a medicinal herb used
by ancient Egyptians and Greeks? Or perhaps it was hydrastis, commonly known as goldenseal, which is widely recognized today as one of
the most popular and effective antibacterial herbs?

The more I became intrigued by this—indeed, by the entire contents of her herbal "medicine chest"—the more I was struck by the

tragedy of it all. Our knowledge of herbal medicine in this country is a direct, wondrous gift from African slaves and early American Indians (Lumbee and Cherokee tribes in particular). Yet millions of Americans today remain profoundly estranged from it.

Call it folk medicine. Call them home remedies. In reality, it's stuff we know if only through oral histories preserved through the ages. It's the chickweed salve our grannies rubbed three layers thick over scars, the garlic brews whipped up for colds, the peach kernels boiled for earaches. Some of us still rely on these things—a quiet nod to ancestors who reveled in the power of nature to heal. This is particularly true of elderly blacks living in the South. Many of them still use herbal medicine as their main source of care or as a supporting treatment. They are put off, says sociologist Wilbur Watson, Ph.D., by the impersonal treatment of the current medical system, with its endless list of doctor referrals and specialists for virtually every organ.

But the use of herbal medicine in American history is, by and large, ignored by the medical establishment. Older African-Americans in the South, as well as those who have lived for decades in racially segregated neighborhoods, depend more on traditions and the wisdom of their elders than on conventional medicine. There is a belief in rural communities that traditional medical practices should not be violated. And there are limits on how much technology will be accepted. Advancements in medical tools and techniques may complement the existing traditional system but not replace it.

The black elderly have purposely shrouded their customs in secrecy for fear of being ridiculed or misunderstood. Similarly, when many of my patients tell other doctors they are seeing a naturopathic physician, they usually receive a snicker, dismissive gesture, or a negative comment. Today in rural North and South Carolina, Louisiana, Georgia, Mississippi, Florida, and Virginia, neighborhood pharmacies with "back rooms" and "spiritual corners" still flourish. Folk remedies are dispensed regularly in these rooms through an informal network maintained by word of mouth.

IGNORING THE PAST

Yet, for most Americans, these are not the traditions that guide health care. When ailment strikes—or bodies give way to the scourge of neglect—more often than not we turn to conventional medical practitioners with their pharmacologic solutions, surgical tools, and scientific preoccupation with symptoms. Even as millions of Americans are eagerly searching for practices such as my own in naturopathy, where I focus on underlying causes of illness as well as the medicinal plants of our past, most Americans still find sanctuary in conventional physicians' offices. Or in none at all.

African-Americans are once again disproportionately represented, or underrepresented, only this time as natural health care consumers, and certainly as practitioners. In my own practice, 65 percent of my patients are white Americans or Europeans, 5 percent are Latinos, and the remaining 30 percent are African-Americans. While nationwide more than one third of all Americans use the services of complementary medical practitioners, in thirty-four out of thirty-five conferences on complementary health care that I have attended, I was the only African-American presenter or participant. And in nearly all of the case studies presented at these conferences, the patients are white.

But how can this be, with African-American history so rich with lessons that now, more than ever, are guiding America's rapidly growing holistic health movement? African slaves, after all, understood healing and medicine in a far deeper way than the allopathic doctors of their time, just as naturopaths and homeopaths understand medicine differently than many of their conventional colleagues today. For Africans, healing always involved not only the person who was ill, but the family, the community, and the interaction among them. Illness was seen as a disharmony between the environment and the patient. Therefore, Africans zealously pursued the causes to determine whether they were natural—that is, created by forces like cold or heat, wind or dampness—or whether they were the result of evil spirits drummed up by conjurers or root doctors—unnatural—or by God as a form of punishment for purported sins.

So it is with naturopaths and homeopaths: We, too, seek the cause of illness. We know wellness is not a solitary venture. We investigate the spiritual, mental, emotional, and physical health of an individual, focusing in particular on the ways in which a patient's lifestyle, habits, and relationships—with family members, coworkers, or neighbors, for example—affect his or her health. Moreover, we don't try to simply kill the pain. We understand that patients don't get headaches from the absence of aspirin, nor are they depressed because of an absence of Prozac.

I see "unnatural" illnesses differently from the way my ancestors did. I believe that they are caused, for example, by negative self-talk and doubt, by judgments against ourselves and others which can result in depression and anxiety. Unlike our ancestors, I do not believe God creates them. We do.

How do we address these troubles once we determine what they are? How did we in the past? Not through conventional medicine. Slave narratives tell us that slaves rejected the medicine given them by their masters' doctors and chose instead familiar remedies from food, roots, and herbs, almost all of which had African origins.

"Oh, de people never didn' put much faith to de doctors in dem days," Josephine Bacchus, an eighty-year-old ex-slave from Marion, South Carolina, recalls in a compilation of slave interviews by historian George Rawick. "Mostly, dey would use de herbs in de fields for dey medicine."

Bacchus proclaims the power of at least two popular roots: black snakeroot and Sampson snakeroot. "Say, if a person never had a good appetite, dey would boil some of dat stuff . . . take a tablespoon of dat bitter medicine three times a day. [I]t bound to swell your appetite." Black snakeroot or cimicifuga (black cohosh) was also used as I use it today, for rheumatism and with other herbs in the treatment of menopause and dysmenorrhea (menstrual cramps).

Her prescription is one of many. In similar narratives by Oklahoma, South Carolina, and Georgia ex-slaves, natural remedies seem to be not only abundant but highly effective. Kiziah Lee, ninety-three, tells us that, when sickness came, "We would take butterfly root and life everlasting and boil it and make a syrup and take it for colds. Balmony and queens delight boiled and mixed would make good blood medicine."

Lou Smith, eighty-three, describes how a tea made out of dog fennel or corn shucks will cure chills. Easter Wells, eighty-three, advises that "Horse mint and palm of crystal and bullnettle root boiled together will make a cure for swelling." Sally Brown notes that jimsonweed was good for rheumatism, chestnut leaf tea for asthma, and "ho-hound" for colds. "[We] made candy out'n it with sorghum molasses." The abolitionist Harriet Tubman was known to use herbs extensively, at one point freely administering them to slave refugees and Union soldiers who fought in the Civil War.

Somehow, between the time of these ex-slaves and now, we turned away from these natural remedies and failed to preserve a tradition that had been passed down through generations, reaching as far back as Africa. Through the history of naturopathy we can see what has gone wrong. We can see what forces have conspired to eat at our knowledge of, and enthusiasm for, the medicines of the past.

In short, modern medicine began to overshadow the good in these traditions. Now in the 1990s we continue to have a skewed perception of medicine in this country. And no wonder. In the past fifty years, we have witnessed major breakthroughs in medicine. Technology has allowed us to diagnose more rapidly and efficiently, and perform life-saving feats.

This is all of great value. But there is a downside.

We now have so many pills and liquids for pain, allergy relief, and suppression of coughs, colds, and influenza that one can hardly keep track. Not to mention antibiotics, antihistamines, antidepressants, antifungals, immunosuppressors, and steroids. We have learned from conventional physicians and the media that, if we are sick, we take a pill that suppresses the condition and kills the germ. Physicians do not teach us to support ourselves and be responsible for our health. We are not taught to support the body's innate ability to heal itself. We are not taught how to prevent illness.

DISTRUST

Ignorance prevents many people from knowing about naturopathy, while poverty prevents them from taking advantage of this healing art. The task is made all the more daunting because many people don't particularly like doctors. Whether allopathic or **naturopathic**, we tend to distrust them. Patients tell me horror stories **about their** health care experiences. Many African-Americans talk about how difficult it is to talk to doctors, particularly white ones, or how quickly white doctors want to perform surgery for insignificant things, often with disastrous results. And I hear many women say how difficult it is to share their problems and concerns with male doctors, regardless of color.

This mistrust is not without historical precedent. For years African-Americans have been treated poorly in the doctor's office, being used and manipulated for research purposes. The notorious Tuskegee syphilis study, which began in the 1930s, is one example of why blacks should be wary of a white-dominated medical industry. U.S. Public Health Services researchers selected dozens of black males to observe the effects of untreated syphilis. Yet in the screening process the white researchers never fully informed their subjects of the painful and damaging results of participating in such a study, and in fact told them they were being treated. For thirty years the study was conducted on over 400 Alabama black men.

When I ask a patient at the beginning of his or her first visit, "Why have you come to me?" and "How would you like homeopathy and naturopathy to help you?" I often hear a variation of one particular patient's response, a man who was taking four different drugs when he came to me.

"I'm here because I want to stay alive," he said. "My doctors are trying to kill me with all these poisons [drugs]. Next they'll tell me I don't need some body part and try to talk me into taking it out."

It is not uncommon in my practice for a patient to be on Mevacor to reduce cholesterol, Catapres to reduce hypertension, Hytrin for enlarged prostate, or Prozac to alleviate depression. These are just a few of the examples of drugs prescribed by allopathic physicians for common ailments. In addition, patients self-medicate with over-the-counter drugs such as antihistamines, without realizing that all drugs have unintended (side) effects. Hytrin, for example, can cause headaches, dizziness, and impotence, the latter two of which this patient experienced.

Such suspicion and mistrust are in part why so many poor people and people of color use emergency rooms as their primary source of medical care. For nonurgent visits the rate for black Americans is almost double the rate for whites. It is no wonder that, when some African-American patients make their way to my office, they have had a condition for five or ten years and sometimes longer; they simply haven't bothered to seek professional assistance. And even then, some who are not well informed have not made the distinction between my work and the work of conventional doctors. They have just heard that I use herbs sometimes. Perhaps, like the ex-slave Mildred Graves, they used herbs extensively at home for much of their lives. To them, I am the "herb doctor," and they are often desperate for help.

But besides our current experiences with conventional medicine, there is another reason behind the doubt and skepticism. It starts with our history of servitude in the United States.

WHITE MEDICINE, BLACK BONDAGE

At the high point of slavery, during the antebellum era, white Southerners owned some four million slaves. It was the labor of these slaves that made white owners wealthy. Yet, because of their unbending belief in white supremacy, whites saw African slaves as a strange species, biologically and genetically different from their own race. Courts vacillated on whether slaves were even human, and numerous court cases supported the idea that they were much like cattle.

In the minds of most whites, then, it followed that blacks had their own peculiar diseases and immunities and that these were distinctly different from their own. But no medical textbook on Negro diseases existed. The illnesses slaves suffered most—cholera, pneumonia, dysentery, yellow fever, and malaria—were due mainly to their living conditions, not their genetic inheritance. Still, whites periodically tried to support this myth with "fact," and the many cure-alls aimed at blacks were the result. Swaim's Panacea, for instance, was touted to cure consumption, or wasting of the body, tuberculosis, feebleness, rheumatism, syphilis, diseases of the liver and skin, and all diseases from impurities of the blood. According to a review published in the 1950s, it was said to be particularly useful for "Negroes who are confined in large numbers on plantations in hot climates."

This interest in special Negro medicine was understandable because the wellness of slaves was critical to the plantation economy and, more generally, Southern agriculture. Without healthy slaves, the economic underpinning of white lives would fall apart.

Still, with all the talk and advertising of special cures, evidence shows that, in practice, blacks generally received the same treatment as whites when they received treatment. This, as it turns out, was not great news for anybody, white or black, as medical care was horridly deficient.

No one knew this better than the slaves themselves, who often avoided revealing illness to their master, lest they be forced to endure "white man's medicine."

Many whites, however, wanted to curtail the rapidly growing number of blacks who called themselves doctors during the 1700s. They refused to acknowledge that there were in fact many qualified black doctors who didn't engage in superstition and quackery. They were also concerned with the increasing number of reports of white owners being poisoned by black doctors. In 1748 the colonial legislature of Virginia prohibited all slaves from administering medicines without the consent of their owners. Slaves who broke the law would be put to death.

There were many efforts to curtail the practice of medicine by blacks throughout the nineteenth century, and though they were generally unsuccessful—because, for one reason, whites sought black doctors anyway—they were examples of how vigilantly whites made certain that African customs and traditions did not flourish.

So legendary was this fear of blacks practicing their own medicine that over the years it found a voice in film and literature. Margaret Walker Alexander's widely celebrated 1966 novel, *Jubilee,* tells of the frightening confrontation the slave girl Vyry had with an overseer and his assistant as she gathered herbs in the swamp. Not only does the scene affirm the varied ways blacks used the earth for their health and survival, it dramatizes to what lengths blacks had to go to claim the right.

"What you doing here by yourself in the swamp woods, Vyry, and what you want with them weeds?"

"Them ain't no weeds, Mister Grimes. Them is greens to cook to eat, and yerbs and roots to cure all kinds of miseries that ails you."

The patter-roller said, "Tell us what you may call 'em and what you makes from them."

"Well, sir this here is my greens. . . . Now that there is mullein. I take mullein and pinetop and salt and I does different nother things with different ones. Mullein bath is good for the feets and legs to stop swelling and heart dropsy. I also uses it for teas. This here is barefoot root. I cooks it down and adds pyo lard and salt and makes a salve for the rheumatiz. Mayapple root is good to work the bowels and black halls and cherry root makes a good tea to strengthen the appetite. Them there is Jerusalem oats for worms. Mosten everybody knows that. . . ."

"You sure you ain't got no pizen [poison] in there, has you?"

"Nossah, I ain't fooling with no pizen. Course I can't tell you what's pizen from what ain't pizen. I just knows the good roots. I ain't never knowed the bad roots."

The truth was, Vyry had successfully hidden her poisonous mushrooms from Grimes. Vyry's mushrooms worked, but many other herbs and roots failed their intended purpose. The result: slaves died or became sicker, and black doctors sometimes found themselves in the same unenviable position as their white counterparts.

Africans were luckier with their practice of midwifery, that gentle art learned in their homeland. As eighty-four-year-old slave Mildred Graves, an active midwife at the time, tells us:

You know in dem days dey didn't have so many doctors. So treatin' de sick was always my job. Whenever any of de white folks 'round Hanover was goin' to have babies dey always got word to Mr. Tinsley dat day want to hire me for dat time. Sho' he lef me go . . . 'twas money fo' him you know. He would give me only a few cents, but dat was kinda good of him to do dat. Plenty niggers was hired out an' didn't get nothing. Sometimes I had three an four sick at de same time. Marser used to tell me I was a valuable slave. Dey used to come fo' me both day an' night—you know it's a funny thing how babies has a way of comin' heah when it's dark.

Midwives attended to the whole woman and the whole process of having a child, not just the baby's delivery from the womb. Slave women excelled in this field, delivering not just their own as they did in Africa, but the babies of plantation wives and overseers. In fact, plantation owners preferred it this way. Because conventional doctors were expensive, slaves were "employed" in an estimated half of the plantation households, usually for little or no money.

There was no doubt that many black herbalists were also on to something, even when stretching their claims. Consider Lydia Pinkham's Vegetable Compound, for which she received a patent in 1875. It contained unicorn root (so named because of its tuberous, cylindrical, and slightly horizontal roots), pleurisy root, life-root, black cohosh, fenugreek seed, and at least 15 percent alcohol. I was fortunate to find an old label of the compound from a druggist in West Virginia. It reads in part:

> It will cure entirely the worst form of Female Complaints, all Ovarian troubles, Inflammation and Ulceration, Falling and Displacements, and the consequent Spinal Weakness, and is particularly adapted to the change of Life. It will dissolve and expel tumors from the uterus in an early stage of development. . . . It removes faintness, flatulency, destroys all craving for stimulants, and relieves weakness of the stomach. It cures Bloating, Headaches, Nervous Prostration, General Debility, Sleeplessness, Depression, and Indigestion.

Obviously Ms. Pinkham's remedy could not live up to all its claims. But as late as the 1980s, African-Americans were still using it and getting various forms of relief, as they were with other compounds such as Humphrey's 11, and black draught, a laxative. I am not surprised. Unicorn root, for instance, is one of the herbs I use today as a uterine and pelvic tonic to assist women through menopause. Pleurisy root is often used to relax muscles and break up congestion, and as an expectorant. Black cohosh, or macrotys, is one of our most useful herbs. It is a stomach tonic that assists with painful intestinal gas as well as menstrual cramps and ovarian pain.

Clearly, naturopathic medicine has been a beneficiary of traditional herbal medicine. In addition to the diseases already mentioned, there are remedies for chicken pox, measles, thrush, and worms. The roots, bark, and leaves of plants from the families of *Allium cepa* and *sativum*, croton, dioscorea, orimum, *Plantago major,* sambucus, sarsaparilla, *Zea mays* all were useful. The landscape and terrain of the Carolinas, Virginia, Georgia, and Louisiana was similar to that of tropical Africa. Today, some of the medicinal plant families are commonly used in my practice or as culinary herbs.

Here's a list of herbs and their historical and current uses:

- **Dioscorea alata,** which is **yam or sweet potato,** was used as an antispasmodic to regulate the bowels. It was also used for the nausea of pregnant women. Now it is used commonly for women who suffer from ovarian or uterine pain during menses.

- **Sambucus canadensis** (American) or **elderberry root** was boiled and used as a tea for bladder infections. **Sambucus nigra** (English) was used for purging the bowel and to create vomiting. Homeopathically it is used for people who complain of thick, tenacious mucus that can create suffocative coughs.

- The **shuck covering of dry corn** or **Zea mays** was used for influenza and colds. Now we use cornstarch for cooking as well as applying it topically for itching and irritations of the skin. Corn silk as a tincture is used for the relief of pain associated with kidney problems as well as a diuretic for the genitourinary tract.

- **Aristolochia serpentaria** or **Virginian snakeroot** was boiled and taken as a tea for infections, viruses, and kidney problems. Today a tea is taken at the onset of a cold to increase circulation and cause sweating. Or serpentaria is an expectorant in tight bronchial coughs. In homeopathy it is indicated for people who suffer from dyspepsia and bloating of the abdomen.

- The bark of the **Prunus serotina** or **Virginia prunus** (wild cherry bark) tree was boiled and taken as a tea for treating asthma. Prepared as a syrup or tincture, today it can be used for reducing mucus discharge and soothing irritated mucous membranes due to bronchitis, a nervous cough, or a simple cold.

- **Boric acid** in an aqueous solution was used as a mouthwash and skin lotion. It is particularly useful as a douche (using one tablespoon of boric acid combined with one quart of warm water) for women in my practice who are suffering from vaginal yeast infections. The douche is to be alternated with acidophilus powder douche; the latter one is given in the morning and the former one is given in the evening.

- **Cimicifuga racemosa, black snakeroot** or **black cohosh** has maintained its usage for rheumatism, and pain and discomfort associated with menstruation. It is used in conjunction with **Caulophyllum (blue cohosh)** and **Mitchella ripens (squawvine)** to produce effectual uterine contractions during labor. The analgesic properties of black cohosh can assist in pleurisy and intercostal neuralgia as well as the discomfort and pain accompanying influenza. Its use in the treatment of menopausal symptoms is also remarkable. The phytoestrogens in this plant exert estrogenic action upon the hormonal system which balances estrogen effects. It also has a vascular effect, thus relieving hot flashes. Historically, it was also a treatment for yellow fever, bronchitis, nervous disorders, and snakebites. In combination with **sarsaparilla (Menispermum canadense)** in corn whiskey, black cohosh was used to treat arthritis and diabetes. Mixed with equal portions of **catnip (Nepeta cataria)** and **wild comfrey (Cynoglossum virginianum)**, the resultant tea was given to seizure patients.

❧ **Chamomile (Anthemis nobilis)**, a very well-known herb, has aided many people in relaxing or getting a good night's sleep. Indigestion and flatulence also respond well to chamomile. Topical applications of the tea were useful for poison ivy and I use the tea in a bath with the liquid from cooked oatmeal to relieve the itching of eczema. (This is also the herb that is used as a design element throughout this book.)

❧ Among the many uses for **Taraxacum officinale** or **dandelion root** is as a mild laxative, antidiabetic diuretic, appetite stimulant, and a digestive aid. Drinking the tea often during a day was also for eczema and scurvy. Its primary use is in kidney and liver disorders as it is a general stimulant and cleanser for these organs. It was used in combination with **white oak bark (Quercus alba)** and **burdock (Arctium minus or lappa)** as a tea for varicose veins.

❧ **Flaxseed** (linseed) or **Linum** has always been and continues to be used as a laxative. Because of its soothing action on irritated mucous membranes (mouth, throat, etc.), pouring boiling water over the seeds makes a drink for coughs. The seeds were also used externally in poultices for skin irritations, burns, and boils.

❧ **Allium sativum,** commonly known as **garlic,** is of course a popular spice as well as a vasomotor depressant. It can, along with exercise and a good diet, reduce essential hypertension. It is also an antibacterial, used topically on boils and pustules and internally to promote sweating during colds and flus. I continue to use it for all of these reasons. In addition it kills intestinal yeast and parasites. Warm garlic oil is very effective in decreasing the pain of ear infections.

❧ **Allium cepa,** the **onion,** also a common condiment, has been used with garlic for colds and flus, boils and abscesses. In Africa it was applied to burns to prevent infection. Crushed onions on the forehead were used for headaches while honey and onion syrup was useful for asthma. For lowering blood cholesterol and blood sugar and reducing the tendency to asthma attacks, onion remains a very useful herb.

❧ **Zingiber officinale Roscoe,** which is **ginger,** was used by the American Indians for heart disorders and to promote menstruation. Now we use it for relief from nausea and vomiting because of its antispasmodic effect. It is also useful in lowering cholesterol.

❧ **Eyebright (Euphrasia officinalis)** was used in the 1800s for watery eyes and dim vision. Its use has changed to include inflammation of the conjunctiva. Equal parts of eyebright, **goldenseal (Hydrastis canadensis),** and **echinacea (Echinacea angustifolia)** are used in distilled water as an effective eye wash.

❧ **White horehound** or **Marrubium vulgare** has always been used for asthma and bronchitis and that hasn't changed. It has also been used to treat diarrhea and kidney ailments. It was a main ingredient in Negro Cezar's antidote for vegetable poisonings.

❧ A very well-known herb is used for everything from candy to colds to menopause—**licorice root** or **Glycyrrhiza glabra.** Its use dates back thousands of years. It is thought to lower the estrogen:progesterone ratio, thus explaining its effect on premenstrual symptoms or PMS. It is used in conjunction with **chaste tree (Vitex agnus castus), black cohosh (Cimicifuga racemosa),** and **dong quai (Angelica sinensis)** as a uterine tonic and as an aid in relieving symptoms of menopause. I use it in my practice almost daily for this reason as well as for the common cold. For a cold I combine licorice with **echinacea, goldenseal,** and **osha root (Ligusticum).** The licorice acts upon the adrenal glands. It increases the half-life of cortisol, which reduces antibody formation, stress reaction, and inflammation, thus increasing the immune function of the body. *Be mindful that if taken in large amounts (in excess of 10 grams of the crude herb) it can cause sodium retention and severe electrolyte imbalance. If you have a history of hypertension or renal failure, consult a physician before taking this herb.*

❧ I also combine **phytolacca** or **poke root** with **echinacea, glycyrrhiza,** and **hydrastis** in a tincture for the treatment of colds with sore throat and swollen glands. As an immune stimulant it acts specifically to increase the activity of white blood cells. As a poultice and in bath water it has been used for skin eruptions, cancerous skin ulcers, and the seven-year itch. Taken internally as well, it is used for any glandular swelling and cystic condition in addition to spasms of the throat. *Large amounts of this herb may be toxic and cause vomiting.*

❧ **Juniper berry (Juniperus communis)** has been used in creams and ointments for eczema and psoriasis. Currently I use this herb in my practice along with **buchu** and **bearberry (Arctostaphylos uva-ursi)** for urinary tract infections. Juniper acts as a diuretic, producing vasodilation of the bladder and kidney.

Conventional medicine, on the other hand, drew a different response from the black population of the day. Most practitioners of this "heroic" medicine, as it was called, followed the pioneering work of Benjamin Rush, a medical doctor and the first chemistry professor in the United States.

Rush earned much of his reputation with one finding: he noticed that increased tension of the arterial system caused most illnesses. He believed the body needed to be purged of impurities that were carried in the blood. With hundreds of doctors following his lead, Rush became a forceful advocate of bloodletting, leeching, and blistering. He also recommended administering substances like antimony and mercury, which, unbeknownst to any of the doctors at the time, were actually poisonous to the human body.

Blacks were particularly suspicious of Rush's approach to medicine. They believed the processes were too harsh. Mary Lindsay, at age ninety-one, recalled in an interview in *The American Slave* (1972) how a visiting doctor dealt with a broken arm. "He say I got bad blood from it how come I git so sick, and he git out his knife out'n his satchel and bleed me in the other arm," she recounted. "The next day he come back and bleed me again two times, and the next day one more time, and then I git so sick I puke and he quit bleeding me."

BREAKING OUT OF BONDAGE

Wary of the medical profession and neglected by their masters, black slaves retained and cultivated their own knowledge of medicinal herbs, roots, and other vegetation. Fortunately for them, the geography and climate of the South closely resembled the slaves' West African homeland, making herbal identification and cultivation of familiar species and families of plants a real possibility. Families passed along what they knew to one another. Indeed, much as in Chinese culture today, where patients go first to herbalists, then acupuncturists, and finally to surgeons, slaves tapped first the resources in their families, then sought out herbalists and midwives, then conjurers (those who called on the spirits), and, only if absolutely necessary, plantation owners and physicians. In Suzanne Terrell's *This Other Kind of Doctor* (1990), one former slave known as "Mama Doc" recalls her mother's approach to medical problems:

She made all kinds of syrups and things for coughs. Her Daddy was half Indian. And you'd take a person that'd be sick an' you know, they don't do now like they did then. Then if a person go sick, an' somebody heard about it, everybody that knowed anything to help anybody would go to them an' do things. An' when they couldn't do what they could do, tried to do, then they'd send get the doctor.

Whites took note because they were keenly aware of the shortcomings of their own doctors. They were inspired to embrace other forms of medicine, but even with a rapid spread of alternative healing practices among whites, the reputation of African blacks as natural healers exceeded both whites and Indians who used herbs. Planters and physicians alike quietly sought them out for advice and care.

In his book *Roll Jordan Roll* (1974), Eugene Genovese remarks how one planter, John Hamilton, of Williamsport, Louisiana, wrote of his conversion in a letter to his brother, a fellow planter. "I am sorry to learn that you have been unfortunate with the Negroes. Your doctors are rather a rough set—they give too much medicine. It is seldom that I call upon a physician. We doctor upon the old woman slave and have first-rate luck."

Fanny Kemble, a planter's wife, is said to have written in her journal about one slave's gift of healing: "I was sorry not to ascertain what leaves she had applied to her ear. These simple remedies, resorted to by savages, and people as ignorant, are generally approved by experience, and sometimes condescendingly adopted by science."

And in an October 1879 issue of Washington, D.C.'s *People's Advocate* newspaper, came this announcement:

NEGRO CEZAR'S CURE FOR THE BITE OF A RATTLESNAKE

Take the roots of plantain or horehound (in summer, roots and branches together), a sufficient quantity, bruise them in a mortar, squeeze out the juice, of which give, as soon as possible, one large spoonful. If the person is swelling, it must be forced down the throat. This generally will cure. If the patient finds no relief in an hour after, give another spoonful which never fails. If the roots are dried, they must be moistened with a little water. To the wound may be applied a leaf of good tobacco, moisten with rum.

Cezar, it turns out, gained his freedom because his herbal remedy for the bite actually worked.

BACKLASH

This is not to say that black doctors—as they were called, though not licensed—were embraced by everyone. Quite the contrary. In one medical journal article after another, slave medicine was routinely blasted as quackery and superstitious nonsense. There was a reason: Slaves also practiced conjuring, voodoo, hoodoo, and witchcraft, and in many cases used them to heal. These forms of black magic and voodoo often overshadowed the helpful work done by herbalists. And even though distinctions clearly existed among conjurers, root doctors, and herbalists, the white population as a whole overlooked them and categorized these groups together. Herbalists, for the most part, didn't want to be associated with "conjurers" or "root doctors" because these practices were typically associated with evil. Herbalists believed their practices were spiritual. Their work, they said, came from God. I agree with Mama Doc, who said, "They was neighborin' people doin' what the Lord tell them to do. What they're doin' is for the advancement of the people. An' they doin' what God wants 'em to do."

These early African-American practitioners were, in many respects, my forerunners. Like me, they used natural substances such as herbs and food to support the body's effort to heal. They treated the whole person, not just the ear or urinary tract or lungs. They pursued the cause of illness, not just the bacterium or virus. And finally, there is one other parallel: Preventive medicine for African slaves was based on personal acts rather than on immunizations or diagnostic tests administered by allopathic doctors. Personal acts are those committed by one person against another. Personal acts also are things we do against ourselves, for example, abuse of drugs (prescription or recreational, including alcohol) or foods, and certainly the abuse of one person by another.

DIET

Herbs played a vital role in the lives of slaves, but it was also their belief in wholesome foods and their practice of midwifery that underscored a genuine understanding of holistic medicine. Though I will explore aspects of diet in later chapters, it is important to mention the role of food now.

In West Africa the diet was simple and nutritious. As far as possible, Africans maintained their customary diet upon coming to America, choosing to eat healthy foods like yams, molasses, sweet potatoes, black-eyed peas, and okra. Yams, for instance, are high in beta carotene and vitamin C, while molasses is high in iron, and black-eyed peas high in fiber. They grew these vegetables whenever they were given the opportunity.

Most of the time, however, Africans ate to survive, having no choice about their diet. Thus, they ate whatever they had: pork, white rice (which has little fiber), white bread, and corn. *Africans did not come here eating salt-laden chitterlings, pigs' feet, hog maws, and fatback.* These unhealthy foods were easy to obtain and allowed them a minimal degree of health. Yet such foods have contributed to the disproportionately high rates of illnesses like hypertension, diabetes, and obesity in the black community. Not only are many of them high in fat and salt content, but these days they are also laced with antibiotics, hormones, and tranquilizers.

Before coming to America, blacks did not suffer from illnesses like respiratory problems, tuberculosis, hypertension, cancer, lactose intolerance, and infectious diseases. But African-Americans continue to suffer from them now as a direct result of the stress of dietary habits and the insufferable living conditions of the slaves.

PAYING HOMAGE

We must follow the ways of our elders. Poverty still is rampant, medical costs continue to skyrocket, and mistrust and lack of rapport continue between patients and medical personnel, particularly between black patients and white professionals and between men and women.

We are as sick now as ever. By the time we come to the attention of health professionals, African-Americans, especially, dominate in categories of severe mental, emotional, and physical symptoms. Today, then, is the time for all of us to reach to the past. Learn from it. Celebrate it. For Americans are not strangers to natural medicine. This is our medicine. This is our heritage. This is our future.

3

HOMEOPATHY

One of the reasons I decided to go to graduate school to study sociology and psychology was that I wanted to have a better understanding of human behavior. I was in my early twenties, fresh out of college and a little naïve about what I wanted to do with my life, although I knew I wanted to "save the world." I had a lot of unanswered questions about the way people acted—the way they responded to things and expressed themselves to one another. I thought that an advanced degree in a field which deals with the interaction of individuals would provide some of these answers.

Long before I made this decision, however, I had always wanted to believe there was more to me than my mind and emotions, my acquisitions and success. No matter how well I did in school, I still felt inadequate. No matter how many friends I made, I still felt separated and distant from them. I needed to make some sense of all the suffering in the world, including my own. I needed to know more about Truth, about the idea that there is something greater than man and his intellect.

I also wanted to rid myself of the sense of inferiority and pain I had accumulated as a black female in this country. I wanted to know more. I wanted to know who I was. I wanted an awareness of myself and how I fit into life. I wanted to understand others so that I might have more compassion and kindness. And I wanted the same for others.

But sociology didn't provide the answers. Nor did my job at the Department of Housing and Urban Development. It wasn't until I began studying natural medicine that I was able to find my true self— and along with that the Truth. As I mentioned in the Introduction, between my second and third year of naturopathic school, while traveling in the Holy Land, I discovered the soul, the part that is connected to the universal spirit that connects to us all. As the New Testament declares, the kingdom of heaven is within us. The true self focuses on the divinity within. It uses love and wisdom to create harmony with God's creations. We are all part of creation. We are made in God's image, and we have the right to be joyful, healthy, and wealthy. We deserve it. This new awareness helped me replace my false self, the self that harbored feelings of fear, insecurity, and pain. This awareness answered my many questions.

The false self is a great force, but not the greatest force. Opposites exist everywhere in nature, including the human psyche. Underneath the negativity of the false self is the positive nature of the true self. Likewise, with homeopathy, the remedies replace the unhealthy patterns and thoughts of the false self with those of the true self. Homeopathic remedies work to eliminate limitations and fixed ideas that make the individual more susceptible to disease.

George Vithoulkas is a world-renowned homeopath and was one of the first Europeans to revitalize homeopathy in North America. About health, in *The Science of Homeopathy,* Mr. Vithoulkas specifically says:

> Health is freedom from pain in the physical body, having attained a state of well-being; freedom from passion on the emotional level, having as a result a dynamic state of serenity and calm; and freedom from selfishness in the mental sphere, having as a result total unification with Truth.

I was intrigued. Going to naturopathic school was a continuation of my search for Truth. I thought homeopathy was a way for myself and my patients to gain freedom and discover the Truth. I was right.

How does all of this talk about God, true self, and false self relate to homeopathy?

Let's begin with an understanding of the mental state. Our mental state is responsible for our memory, concentration, and creativity, among other things. A mental disturbance comes in a variety of different conditions and refers to more than just medical diagnoses like schizophrenia or manic depression. For example, a mental disturbance may make it difficult to express one's thoughts or to find the right word in conversation.

A mental disturbance may also hinder your consciousness. When you begin to lose awareness of yourself in relationship to others and the environment, the result is harmful behavior like selfishness or greed. Self-absorption and intolerance are other signs of this mental disturbance. We cannot know the Truth when we are operating out of self-advancement and egotism. Instead, we become oblivious to others' needs.

We usually know when we are mentally healthy. We are aware of being part of a greater whole. Our behavior is likely to be productive and fruitful. We pursue goals of health, happiness, wealth, and love. We encourage others to do the same. We have selfless creativity for ourselves and others. When we are well, we can give freely of ourselves, from the overflow of who we are. When we are well, it hurts *not* to give.

Emotional wellness requires the ability to feel. When patients say they have no feeling about a situation or life experience, I find they have likely suppressed the feeling or disassociated from it because it is too painful. In order to survive emotionally, these patients have had to separate themselves from the experience, as if it happened to someone else. There is an Ethiopian proverb, "He who conceals his disease cannot expect to be cured." We should try not to hide that which is making us sick. Also, when we react to things in the past, we are unable to deal with things in the present and therefore become emotionally unhealthy. We need to be able to feel the range of emotions, from good to bad, to be healthy. When we have emotional freedom, we are able to experience our feelings and let go of them. We don't burden ourselves with one emotion. We become angry, for example, but it is an anger that is appropriate in degree and intensity for that situation. Emotional freedom enables us to return to a state of peace and calm.

On the other hand, physical health is much easier to assess. We are used to focusing on our physical condition when we are sick. Physicians have grown accustomed to focusing on physical disease, picking out individual organs to heal rather than the entire person. In fact, the medical establishment was so intent on dealing with physical symptoms, it did not recognize a connection between mind and body until recently. Yet most people would admit that conditions like fatigue, chronic headaches, or arthritis are closely connected to our emotional state. Physical health allows us to be energetic and pain-free and to experience a state of well-being.

Now, having a greater understanding of wellness and homeopathy, I believe it is the one medicine that touches deeply into a person, truly creating wellness on all levels, for the homeopathic remedies touch the soul.

Treating the Whole Person:
Body, Mind, and Soul—An Acute Condition

Whether we believe a condition like arthritic pain makes one irritable and angry, or whether an angry and irritable nature contributes to arthritic pain, we cannot deny the connection between our natures and our bodies. Homeopaths view the person and the symptoms in a totality; and it is the totality of symptoms in a person that we treat. The homeopath will individualize a treatment by assessing the state and the nature of the patient in order to give the correct remedy. However, there are times when the physical symptoms are so overwhelming that they must be the focus for a homeopath. Following is an example of when a homeopath recognizes a patient's acute condition.

Not long ago a patient named Patricia called to say she thought the cold she had had for the past week was moving into her lungs. She felt weak and exhausted and had spiking fevers of 104 degrees. During our conversation I noted a hard, dry cough she said was painful. She had aches all over her back, but particularly in an area just above her kidneys. Even the slightest movement increased the pain in this area. While normally a loving and active mother with three children, Patricia was extremely irritable because of her illness. She had barely eaten over the past few days, and complained of an intense and chronic thirst.

It was clear from the symptoms that Patricia's neglected cold had developed into pneumonia.

Homeopaths do not have one remedy for this condition. We have many remedies for people who have pneumonia. One of the options, bryonia (a plant known as wild hops), seemed to fit all of the patient's physical and emotional symptoms. I prescribed the remedy bryonia in 1M potency, which means the herbal tincture of bryonia was a 1:1000

(M) dilution and then diluted one more time (1)1.* By the next day the patient was appreciably better. I repeated the bryonia 1M the third day and within the next week she was cheerful and healthy once again. Also on the third day, I prepared an herbal tincture of grindelia, lobelia, glycyrrhiza, phytolacca, and echinacea to be taken in 30-drop doses, four times a day. This combination of herbs acts as an immune stimulant, an antiviral, and an expectorant. Had her symptoms not been resolved by the third day, I would have referred her to a medical doctor for antibiotics.

If Patricia had exhibited other symptoms with the pneumonia, I would have prescribed a different remedy. If, for instance, she wept frequently, craved affection and attention, and was thirstless, I would have prescribed pulsatilla rather than bryonia. Like any homeopath, I adjusted the treatment according to the patient's needs. Her story is an example of an acute condition that requires an understanding of the person's nature in order to determine the correct remedy.

TREATING THE WHOLE PERSON:
MIND, BODY, AND SOUL—A CHRONIC CONDITION

For homeopaths, chronic conditions are similar to acute ones. We must understand the patient in order to find the right remedy. Classical homeopaths are resolved to assist patients to be in harmony with the universe, to reestablish them in a partnership with themselves and with their God. We are vehicles through which God offers positive rather than negative energy, light rather than darkness.

My first visit with a new patient lasts at least an hour and a half. This is a time when I have an opportunity to understand who the patient is: his or her fears, grief, anxieties—past and present—and the patient's goals and hopes for the future. Whatever patients remember to tell me during the interview is typically what is most important to them or what is affecting them the most. It is a time when I am listening, not advising or directing, but just being with them. For many patients, it is a time to share concerns or feelings about themselves that they have never voiced

---

*Unless you are a physician, you probably cannot get this potency. If you believe, based on your reading, that you need Bryonia, take whatever potency you have and call a physician who can assist you.

before. Sometimes they cry as they have never cried before. It can be a cathartic time.

Because there are many remedies for fear and grief and because homeopaths individualize the treatment for every patient, it is critical for the homeopath to know as much about the person's history as possible. The history brings me closer to understanding the disease state: a state adopted by the person for survival in a particular situation, a function in response to a sensation, a constriction or a band that forms around the person.

I recall the case of a fifty-year-old patient who came into my office complaining of lethargy, anemia, and allergies. She was medicated on nasal sprays, antihistamines, and an antidepressant. She also took decongestants even though they made her anxious. She required lots of sleep and still had low energy.

"My body shuts down, closes down on me," she told me. "I feel it. Then I feel sick."

Michelle had suffered from allergies and eczema since she was a baby. Her condition was so bad as a child that her parents had to put gloves on her hands to keep her from scratching herself. She had received allergy shots, on and off, for many years. But whenever she went off the shots, she was prone to get nasty, lingering colds.

After explaining that there are many remedies for allergies and fatigue, and that the goal in my office is to treat people, not conditions, I asked her to tell me about herself: her nature, mood, and the challenges in her life. The story that unfolded was filled with pain and suffering, both physical and emotional. Once she finished describing her life, I had no doubt why she was sick.

Michelle was the youngest of four children and the only daughter in the family. One of her brothers was diagnosed with diabetes at an early age and received her mother's constant attention. Another brother, the oldest, was without question her mother's favorite, a fact that her mother would admit to friends even in front of the other children. Michelle had an absentee father who spent most of his time drinking with friends. He would leave the house on Friday and not come back until Sunday evening. It wasn't until Michelle was sixteen, when her father hit her mother for the first and last time, that he was finally asked to leave.

For much of her childhood Michelle felt rejected and unloved, as if her needs and desires were not important. As she grew older, that didn't change. She worked at a department store to save money for college, despite the fact that her mother wanted the oldest son to go to school instead. For her mother, it wasn't enough that Michelle wanted to go, or that both of these children, if they so desired, could go to college. It was more important that the oldest son have a better opportunity than the rest of the kids.

When Michelle was ten, the brother closest to her was killed in a car accident. He was crossing the road after being dropped off by the school bus. The driver had no chance of seeing him. Michelle was devastated. She turned to other family members for support, but neither her mother nor her two other brothers could help. They had shut themselves down emotionally to deal with the tragedy.

As she spoke to me about her brother's death, Michelle recalled times when she and her brother would play in the house after school. Sometimes they would make cardboard toys out of cereal boxes, or play practical jokes on other kids in the neighborhood. One time, when Michelle cut herself in the head playing on a swing, her brother sprinted all the way home to get their mother. It was just a slight cut, but her brother was convinced she was going to bleed to death and hurried home as fast as he could. It showed how much he cared about her.

Michelle began to cry as she told me these stories. It had been years since she had thought about these memories of her brother, she admitted to me.

With tears flowing down her cheeks, Michelle told me she wasn't good at expressing her feelings to other people. She talked only after she felt comfortable with people. She needed to feel accepted in order to talk; she needed to know that people had a desire to be with her. She would introduce herself to people again and again because she didn't think she was interesting enough to be remembered. She felt ashamed that no one took the time to groom her. No one taught her manners or social graces. She never knew how to interact at a party. She was often left out of group activities. She was also self-conscious about her appearance. She worried that her dark skin and short hair made her unappealing.

Michelle often internalized her feelings because she had few people in life to share them with. At the slightest hint of rejection, she would shut down and deny her feelings. Her introversion was perceived as aloofness. It was a defense mechanism that protected her from being hurt.

Her ex-husband was an angry and negative person who demanded a lot of her attention. He drained her emotionally. A few months after their wedding, Michelle could no longer take his demanding nature and withdrew from him emotionally. She stopped confiding in him. In response, he turned to other people for attention. He began to date other women and stayed out late at night. They had been separated for three and a half years and were now in the process of getting a divorce.

On a physical level, Michelle also had problems. She was about twenty pounds overweight, and she moved her bowels only every other day even with Metamucil. Her long-term memory was not good and her short-term memory was only fair, though her concentration seemed fine. She craved salty foods, chocolate, and wine.

By the end of our first session I knew Michelle was an intelligent, capable woman, but someone who had suffered tremendous grief. It was clear that the source of this grief dated back to her childhood, from experiencing the death of her brother to the neglect by both her parents, but especially her mother. And from this grief arose feelings of insecurity and distrust. Michelle's failed marriage and her belief that she was unattractive only compounded these feelings. As a result, Michelle had built a wall, or shield, around her so that she would not be vulnerable to being hurt ever again. She was sensitive, not aloof, and very responsible. She became academically accomplished at an early age by using her emotional energy to study and by suppressing her emotions through her involvement in school.

Remember the comment about the body shutting down? All of Michelle's bodies—mental, emotional, physical—shut down. It was clear that, though the source of grief dated to a time in her youth, she was brooding and agonizing over the circumstances. In her current condition, she was not free to fully experience other emotions, to fully experience physical or spiritual well-being. I prescribed the remedy natrum muriaticum 200 c for lethargy, anemia, and depression.

Three weeks after our initial visit, she returned to the office to see one of my assistants, who instructed her on my detoxification diet. The diet was to be followed for a ten-day period after which she returned to see me. Upon her third visit, I gave her a diet based on her blood type. (The detoxification process and diets for blood types are explained in

Chapter 4.) Six weeks after her first visit she reported feeling much better. She had stopped all over-the-counter medication and took herself off the antidepressant. Her sleep, energy level, and mood were much improved.

"I feel like myself," she said. "I feel like a normal person."

Four months later she returned for a checkup. Her divorce was final. She said she cried a lot because of it but was not depressed. After a hard campaign, she was elected as an officer of a national organization. She was offered a job in another state but turned it down. She now had several job offers for local consulting positions, but she turned all of them down and was developing a career as a writer and researcher. She was still feeling well.

How does homeopathy bring about wellness for someone like Michelle? How is it that the remedy natrum muriaticum (chloride of sodium) could have possibly created mental, emotional, and physical changes in the patient? How do we know what remedy to choose from the hundreds of remedies we have for "depression" or "allergies"? These answers are the essence of homeopathy.

DR. HAHNEMANN AND THE VITAL FORCE

The term "the healing power of nature" (vis medicatrix naturae) was first voiced by Hippocrates, the father of medicine. More than any other healing art of naturopathic medicine, homeopathy is founded upon this philosophy. Homeopathic remedies are made from plant, mineral, chemical, animal, and insect kingdoms. At the core of this philosophy is vitalism (as described in Chapter 1), or the belief that there is an unknowable inner essence, an energy which animates everything we call life. It is the individualized spirit, the vital force, the soul.

The soul is the force that comes into us at the time of conception and leaves our body at the time of our death. It is that which makes us breathe. Hold your breath for as long as you can and you will see how the vital force forces you to breathe. It coordinates bodily functions so that we may survive in varying environments and changing conditions. It regulates the processes involved in health and disease, gives life and energy to our emotions, and allows us to have thought and reasoning abilities. It connects each of us to one another and to the universe.

The defense mechanism is part of the vital force that acts specifically to maintain balance in the body. When the stimuli are ordinary and routine, we are not aware of any changes in the vital force. But if a stimulus is stronger than the vital force, an imbalance is created that causes the defense mechanism to produce signs and symptoms. We are accustomed to calling groups of these symptoms "diseases," when actually they are the results of the organism's attempt to defend itself and maintain balance. We are also accustomed to thinking we have many "diseases." We do not. Each of us has one "disease" in our body with many signs and symptoms. It is the entire being that is involved in the disease or healing process. Effective therapy should cooperate with the response of the vital force and should treat the entire being, not just a single symptom, organ, or "disease."

Dr. Samuel Hahnemann (1755–1843), the founder of homeopathy, understood that without the vital force the functions of the body could not remain in balance; its sensations and feelings would be absent. He believed that all things in nature were to be used, along with responsibility and compassion, for healing humanity. He combined his understanding of vitalism with the Hippocratic oath, which says in part, "First do no harm." Using natural therapies for healing was his intention and it was to be accomplished rapidly and gently; the disease was to be removed in the least harmful way.

Hahnemann was highly respected for his knowledge of medicine, pharmacology, and chemistry. Soon after he began studying medicine, he became disillusioned with the field. The healing methods being used in the medical programs advocated purging, blistering, and bloodletting, methods which usually exacerbated, not healed, the patient's sickness. In 1782 he left the practice of medicine so that he might "no longer incur the risk of doing injury."

Homeopathic Provings

Hahnemann's quest for knowledge enabled him to discover and systematize the laws of cure relevant to homeopathy. While translating medical books, he began to challenge his colleagues on their findings: specifically, that cinchona was effective against malaria and fevers because of its bitter and astringent qualities. Hahnemann disagreed and decided to take cinchona (Peruvian bark) himself and note the effects. After taking ½ ounce four times a day for several days, he began to experience the symptoms characteristic of malarial fever. His extremities became cold and he felt drowsy. He had heart palpitations and a weak pulse. He experienced anxiety, prostration, and trembling of the limbs, redness of the cheeks, and an insatiable thirst. The sensation of numbness and dullness of mind accompanied all of these symptoms. When he discontinued the herb, he became symptom-free. Only when he repeated a dose did the symptoms return.

From this experience Hahnemann realized that a substance that can produce signs and symptoms in a well person can cure someone with the same symptoms. A root that produces fevers in a healthy individual can work to eliminate fevers in a sick one. This principle, known as the Law of Similars, or let like be treated by like, was first recognized by Hippocrates, who noted that herbs given in toxic doses created the same symptoms they cured when given in low doses.

But Hahnemann also recognized the importance of human experimentation. Healthy subjects were given a material in high enough concentration to disturb their well-being and stimulate their defense mechanism. The body's (vital force) response to this foreign substance was the most intelligent response it could make at the moment, and that response was known as symptoms. This systematic process of testing substances on healthy people is called "proving."

These observations made it clear to him that every medicinal substance (herb, mineral, etc.) alters the mental, emotional, and physical state of a healthy person in a different way. When symptoms were produced as a result of this reaction, he and his assistants laboriously recorded every alteration in the person, every observation in detail, paying special attention to those characteristics that were individualizing to or specific to the person. These observations reflected the curative potential of the substance.

Because of the impressive results of clinical trials treating mental, emotional, and physical conditions, homeopathy became popular by the mid-nineteenth century. It was especially well received because of its effectiveness against scarlet and yellow fever, malaria, cholera, and typhoid.

The details of these experiments and observations are recorded in homeopathic texts which have descriptions of symptoms that result when healthy people take a particular substance. Each substance and its associated symptoms are listed.

Thanks to these textbooks, homeopaths can discern the exact remedy for a person. *The Encyclopedia of Pure Materia Medica,* by Dr. T. F. Allen, gives the following description of the effect of natrum muriaticum, the same medication given to my patient Michelle:

> She was involuntarily obliged to weep. If only one looked at him, he was obliged to weep. Sad and depressed. Depression of spirits. Melancholy mood; she has preferred to be alone for several days past. The more he was consoled the more he was affected. If she only thinks of a want long since past, tears come into her eyes. Always in his thoughts he seemed to seek for past unpleasant occurrences, in order to think them over, making himself morbid. Full of grief; he tormented himself; he seemed to prefer disagreeable thought, which prostrated him very much.

Another modern text, by Roger Morrison, lists similar characteristics of a patient who should be prescribed natrum muriaticum. These characteristics include:

- ❧ Closed, responsible, dignified, and much affected by grief.
- ❧ Ailments from grief and disappointed love. Silent grief.
- ❧ Too serious and overly proper and responsible.
- ❧ Easily offended or wounded; complains of humiliation.
- ❧ Aversion to company.
- ❧ Dwells on past grief and humiliation.
- ❧ Fastidious. Perfectionist. Compulsive.
- ❧ Averse to consolation.
- ❧ Fear. Fear of robbers, the dark, storms, insects, germs, heights.

Homeopaths continue to conduct provings with substances in their raw form or in a potentized form (potentization will be defined later; see p. 55). Within the past year I have personally participated in provings of yellow rose and dolphin's milk, just to name two.

POTENTIZATION AND MINIMUM DOSE

All matter is surrounded by or made up of an electromagnetic field. This field is invisible to the naked eye, but we are able to see it with the help of instruments. Earth, for example, is surrounded by a powerful electromagnetic field known as the Van Allen belts, two zones of high-intensity radioactive fields that extend a thousand miles into space. The human body also has its own energy field. Through the use of Kirlian photography, a technique developed by Soviet scientists in the 1960s, we are able to see energy in the form of a brilliant circle of colors and shadings around an individual. Medical experiments with Kirlian photography have shown that patients who suffer from a disease will emit different forms of color and light. Sometimes a disease will appear in the photography long before it manifests itself in the physical body. A material substance, even the human body, is essentially intense or solid energy.

The vital force is the electromagnetic field of the human body. When a person is exposed to a stimulus, whether good or bad, the energy of the vital force changes. For instance, the death of a loved one induces a stimulus of grief. This change occurs on the mental and emotional level first and may lead to physical alterations. Exposure to a bacterium or virus alters the physical level first and then may alter the mental and emotional level. The person may eventually suffer from poor concentration and irritability or, in the case of fever, hallucinations.

Dr. Hahnemann understood that, in order to affect the vital force, a substance's energy must be compatible with that of the vital force. He knew he had to provide energy to the defense mechanism to help it maintain balance and wellness. Because the only manifestation of the defense mechanism takes the form of signs and symptoms, the healing substance had to produce those same signs and symptoms.

Hahnemann used his provings to determine which substances would match the same signs and symptoms exhibited by the defense mechanism at the time of disease. But he had to find a way to lower the concentration of the material substance to avoid getting the patient sick. He knew he had to weaken the material substance. Dilution alone did not serve his purpose. It weakened the substance to the point where it no longer made the patient sick, but it also weakened the substance's valuable healing effects.

Finally, after months of trial and error, Hahnemann discovered that, by *succussing* (shaking) the diluted material, he could increase the material's intensity and make the same quantity more available to the defense mechanism. This process of dilution and succussion is called *potentization*. A substance that was diluted and succussed produced greater therapeutic results and had less toxic risk.

An example of a succussed homeopathic remedy is the natrum muriaticum 200 c given to Michelle. The "c" is a symbol for a centesimal scale (dividing or diluting something in a ratio of 1:100). The material substance (chloride of sodium) is dissolved in an alcohol and water solution. The mixture stands for two weeks in a dark place and is periodically agitated. The mixture is then strained in a machine to separate the liquid from the material and the subsequent solution is called a tincture. One drop of that tincture is put into 99 drops of an alcohol and water solution and succussed 100 times, usually by a special machine, though sometimes it is done by hand. This process is repeated 200 times. What remains after this process is the essence of natrum muriaticum. It is that essence that was given to the patient.

How Does Homeopathy Work?

It is unclear how the medicinal properties of natrum muriaticum or any other substance are transmitted to the liquid in which it is dissolved. Homeopaths believe that in some way the energy in the original substance gets imprinted onto the liquid molecules and those molecules take on the energy or essence of the original substance. This theory has been verified repeatedly by European researchers.

Once the homeopathic remedy is administered to a patient, it elicits a reaction from the vital force to make the actual physical, mental, and emotional changes necessary for healing the organism. Hahnemann wrote about how the vital force responds to the homeopathic remedy. He based the reaction on natural law. A weaker energy influence in the human organism is permanently destroyed by a stronger one which resembles it in expression. When the vital force, which has been disturbed, is influenced by the stronger artificial agent of potentized medicine, the disease created by the weaker agent disappears. In other words, you have two diseases trying to exist in the organism: one of them is created by a plant or mineral or animal substance (the remedy) and the other is created by a stress—something physical or emotional. The stronger, artificial agent takes hold of the vital force, and the person gets well again.

It is clear that psychic and physical influences do not always have the power to harm our bodies. We become ill because of our susceptibility. But Hahnemann noted every medicine can always affect every living organism and create particular symptoms. Every person can be affected by a medicinal disease, such as the way chloride of sodium affected healthy people in the provings. So the medicinal diseases need to have a stronger influence than natural ones. The medicinal force takes over those parts of the organism that the weaker force was affecting.

Is Homeopathy a Placebo?

In a word, no. The remedy either works or it doesn't. That is not to say that there is not an influence that pacifies the patient. There is potential for a placebo effect because of the relationship established between the doctor and the patient during the initial interview. The doctor's purpose is to be with the patient, to listen, observe, and learn about the patient's personal, family, and medical history. Other variables that influence the healing process may be the patient's fears and distrust of conventional medical practices, or his interest in the mind/body connection.

But if the placebo effect were the only reason a person's health improves, homeopathy would not work on infants, toddlers, children, and animals. But homeopathic remedies *do* work on these patients. It is true, whether we are treating an animal, child, or adult, we might need three or four visits and give the same number of remedies before we see consistent improvement. This happens if we don't understand the patient after the first interview or because the patient has had so much emotional trauma in life. And remedies, unlike placebos, often aggravate the symptoms before alleviating them.

Because homeopathy treats individuals and not diseases, it is difficult to test the value of homeopathic remedies. People with the same diseases will receive different remedies, thus complicating research to narrow a single remedy for a specific disease. But researchers at least have been able to test the effectiveness of specific homeopathic treatments on a particular set of symptoms. Under such a study, the patients are divided randomly into groups, but only one group is actually given the prescribed remedies; the others are given placebos.

Several studies have demonstrated the efficacy of homeopathy using this method, two of which were published recently in *Pediatrics* and the prestigious British medical journal, *The Lancet.* But additional research is necessary to satisfy the most strident critics. I know, however, that when a patient is given the correct remedy homeopathy works. And homeopathy works in a natural way, the way the body intended to cure itself of ailments.

Thanks to the pioneering work of people like Hahnemann and the new material being proven among classical homeopaths, my colleagues and I have a vast body of knowledge to build from. We no longer ask ourselves the question of whether homeopathy works. We ask ourselves what substance in the universe this patient needs at this time. We are developing new provings and new solutions for a broader spectrum of patients and a broader spectrum of diseases.

4

NUTRITION AND YOUR BLOOD TYPE

The doctor of the future will give no medicine but will interest his patients in the care of the human frame, in proper diet, and in the cause and prevention of disease.

—*Thomas A. Edison*

Food is medicine. Hippocrates said, "Let food be thy medicine and medicine thy food." Never has this statement been more important than today, as we witness the emergence of so many long-term chronic illnesses that could have been avoided with proper nutrition. Diseases such as arthritis, diabetes, hypertension, obesity, and cancer (breast, colon, and prostate) are examples of conditions tied to poor nutrition.

Eating well means eating foods that support our bodies, particularly our bodies' cells. Whether those cells make up organs and tissues, or control respiration or digestion, they essentially have the same needs we do: to ingest nutrients and eliminate waste. Because weakened cells have less resistance to disease, one's health depends on the condition of one's cells. So it is important to know the ways in which foods affect our cells. For example, nerve and muscle cells need daily amounts of calcium and vitamin B.

Because we often shortchange our bodies of proper nutrition, our cells become extremely susceptible to disease. And while we have come a long way from the early 1980s, when in one year each average American consumed 100 pounds of refined sugar, 55 pounds of fat and oils, 300 cans of soda, 18 pounds of candy, 5 pounds of potato chips, 7 pounds of corn chips, popcorn, and pretzels, and 50 pounds of cakes and cookies, we still continue to eat alarming amounts of junk food. In 1996 the per capita consumption of refined sugar was 67 pounds, considerably lower than the previous figure but still not anywhere in an ideal range. As a result of eating so much junk food, we have inhibited the body's ability to heal itself or prevent illness. Add this to the other dietary favorites of African-Americans, such as "soul food" and fried food, and we can begin to see how our susceptibility to disease may be magnified. These foods cause stress.

SUGAR

There is no doubt refined sugar is probably the single most dangerous and frequently consumed food for my patients—and for most Americans. It has been responsible for hyperactive, schizophrenic, and violent behavior. But it also has long-term damaging effects on the body. Produced by a chemical process from the sugar cane or sugar beet, sugar has no fiber or nutrients. Most people recognize that sodas, cakes, cookies, candy, and ice cream all contain large amounts of sugar in different forms (fructose, dextrose, corn syrup, and malt). But people must also remember that sugar can be found in cereals, canned soups and vegetables, ketchup, mustard, salad dressings, mayonnaise, processed meats, and even tobacco.

Refined white sugar is harmful to our systems because it does not get digested in the mouth or stomach. It passes directly to the intestines, where it becomes predigested glucose and then is absorbed directly into the bloodstream. There it disturbs the delicate balance of oxygen and glucose in the body. The brain, which relies on consistent sugar levels to function properly, becomes aware of the sugar-level imbalance and tries to compensate by producing adrenal hormones. This is why a three o'clock chocolate bar picks us up temporarily but eventually gives us a tired, listless, and irritable feeling, thanks to the influx of adrenal hormones.

Refined sugar is high in calories. It has no nutritional value, and it robs the body of nutrients like vitamins C and B, chromium and other minerals necessary to metabolize sugar. The body, for example, will draw calcium from the bones and teeth to protect and buffer the blood from excessive sugar levels. Sugar also lowers the body's ability to fight infection by decreasing the function of white blood cells, which play a vital part in the body's immune system. Sugar reduces the body's ability to produce antibodies, which help the body fight against viruses and bacteria.

Some recent studies suggest that sugar may also cause some of the deadliest diseases discussed later in this book. High levels of insulin, the hormone produced when sugar is eaten, contribute to the development of diabetes, obesity, high blood pressure, high triglyceride levels, and low levels of the "good cholesterol," HDL. There are also studies that report that cancerous cells feed on glucose, thus increasing the risk of tumorous cell growth.

CAFFEINE

Caffeine is the world's most popular drug. Four out of five Americans drink it daily. Initially it is a stimulant, reaching peak concentrations in the bloodstream within thirty to sixty minutes. Its secondary reaction, however, is to be a depressant, taking four to six hours for its effect to wear off. During the phase of stimulation it heightens concentration, creates anxiety, and gives us the appearance of more energy. It interferes with sleep and increases blood pressure temporarily. As a depressant, it leaves us fatigued and groggy, with an inability to decipher complex word problems or complicated tasks. This is fairly common knowledge but the effects that we don't often hear about include the following:

- ❧ Caffeine increases the likelihood of osteoporosis because, for example, the more caffeinated coffee one drinks the more calcium leaves the bone and is excreted in the urine.
- ❧ The higher the number of milligrams of caffeine taken during pregnancy, the more likely a woman is to deliver a low-birth-weight baby. Lower birth weight means increased risk of disease and death during infancy.
- ❧ The risk of miscarriage is increased as a woman increases her consumption of caffeine. And pregnancy is less likely for women drinking just one cup of coffee a day.
- ❧ Caffeine is addictive. Coffee accounts for three quarters of the caffeine we consume. But caffeine is in everything from

citrus sodas (orange, lemon-lime), colas, and chocolate to aspirin.

OTHER POISONS

Of course, sugar and caffeine aren't the only poisons we ingest under the guise of food. MSG (monosodium glutamate), a form of salt used to preserve foods and disguise inferior food quality, contributes to numerous health problems. MSG occurs naturally in some foods like Roquefort cheese, milk, tomato, orange juice. It is used in milk and nut products and soups, and can be found in animal feed because it induces cattle, pigs, poultry, and sheep to eat more. In humans, it can cause gastric distress such as belching and bloating, headache, numbness, weakness, and palpitations.

Sodium nitrate and sodium nitrite, used to make meat look brighter and fresher, can produce carcinogenic, mutagenic, and teratogenic changes in the body, and can cause an asphyxiating disease in infants. They can also induce arthritic symptoms and decrease liver storage of vitamin A and carotene, which lead to deficiency symptoms.

In addition to these chemical preservatives, tranquilizers, antibiotics, and hormones injected into live cattle and poultry harm our bodies as well. Tranquilizers calm the animals. Antibiotics prevent diseases from spreading in the overcrowded living conditions. Hormones make the animals develop faster. Meat laced with these chemicals leaves our cells susceptible to any disease to which we may have a familial predisposition (hypertension, diabetes, cancer, arthritis, etc.). For women, hormones found in meat can increase sexual development and cause fibroid tumors.

Butylated hydroxyanisole (BHA) and butylated hydroxytoluene (BHT) are two other popular preservatives. BHA and BHT are banned in Japan, Sweden, and Australia because they have been found to cause liver cancer in rats. Originally developed to prevent color film from deteriorating, BHT can be found in many popular dry foods, including crackers, packaged nuts, cereals, gelatins, puddings, and pie fillings. In humans, BHT has produced low growth rate, loss of weight, liver and kidney damage, increased serum cholesterol, baldness, fetal abnormalities, extreme weakness, fatigue, edema, difficult breathing, and severe allergies. BHT is more toxic and less expensive than BHA.

And let's not forget food dyes—particularly yellow—made from tartrazine, which can be found in jams, cheddar cheese, cheese puffs, some butters, candies, and cakes. This chemical triggers asthma attacks and hives, both of which can be deadly.

How can our cells survive under the pressure of these poisons? They cannot. This is why I guide my patients on how to eat well. At the end of the first appointment, the homeopathic interview, I ask patients to record the foods they eat for five consecutive days along with their bowel and urine habits. Most patients are shocked when they realize what they consume daily—both quantity and quality—and how irregularly they defecate. If you eat daily you should defecate *daily*. Until my patients record their diets for this period of time, it is difficult for them to see how diet can create diseases like arthritis, allergies, diabetes, headaches, heart disease, especially if they do not have digestive problems and believe they can eat anything. What follows is a patient diet diary typical of many:

DAY 1

noodles and vegetables	8:30 A.M.
pear	3:00 P.M.
pasta and sauce	7:00 P.M.
nachos and salsa	12:00 midnight

DAY 2

nonfat milk and a bagel	8:30 A.M.
chicken breast	2:00 P.M.
noodles, vegetable and tuna	8:00 P.M.
popcorn and peanuts	11:00 P.M.

DAY 3

bagel and low-fat cream cheese	9:00 A.M.
beef, potato and vegetable soup and chicken breast	12:00 P.M.
potato chips	2:00 P.M.
chicken and noodles microwave dinner	7:00 P.M.
No bowel movement	

Day 4
½ chicken breast	8:30 A.M.
potato chips, nachos and salsa	6:00 P.M.
chicken and noodles microwave dinner	7:00 P.M.
hummus and pita bread	11:00 P.M.

Day 5
bacon cheeseburger	11:00 A.M.
pear	6:00 P.M.
fried chicken (carry out)	8:00 P.M.
No bowel movement	

This patient commented that he had made a concerted effort not to eat sugar this week. Normally he ate something sweet two or three times a day.

Let's look at another diet diary:

Day 1
oatmeal, white toast, orange juice	9:00 A.M.
chicken noodle soup and white flour crackers	7:00 P.M.

Day 2
fish and collard greens	
macaroni and cheese, candy	4:00 P.M.
No bowel movement	

Day 3
tomato soup, pot roast	3:00 P.M.
ice cream and cake	4:00 P.M.

Day 4
grits, ham, orange juice	8:00 A.M.
fish, pork and beans	4:00 P.M.
No bowel movement	

During their second visit, I explain to patients how diets like those listed above do not support their cells. These foods do not provide proper nutrients for organ systems to be able to defend against disease.

There are several reasons for this statement. Many of these foods are processed (refined white flour, sugar, or rice) and have preservatives, such as the ones mentioned earlier. Also, the salt content of these diets is generally high. Bacon and ham, while high in fat and salt, also have nitrates, essentially another poison to the body. And all the commercial meats eaten in these diets are full of the antibiotics, hormones, and toxins discussed previously.

MILK

We also talk about dairy products, especially milk. Scientific research has linked certain health risks with cow's milk because of the proteins, fats, sugar, and contaminants in milk. In fact, the American Academy of Pediatrics recommends that infants under a year of age not drink whole milk, because of the excessive amounts of contaminants found in an average store-bought carton of whole milk. The use of cow's milk can cause blood loss through the stool, perhaps due to allergic reactions to the proteins in milk. Also, in 1992, the *New England Journal of Medicine* reported that the combination of a genetic predisposition and drinking of cow's milk may be one of the major causes of childhood diabetes.

Milk is also one of the most common causes of problems related to food allergies. Many people of color know that reactions to milk are due to the absence of lactase, the enzyme in our stomach that digests milk sugar, lactose. Be aware that if you can digest milk the lactose breaks down into glucose and galactose, the latter of which has been found to contribute to cataracts and ovarian cancer. Our inability to digest milk (diarrhea and gas) is only part of the problem. Milk proteins, which should be broken down into individual amino acids by the stomach digestive juices (acids), also appear as antigens farther down the intestinal tract and may cause allergic reactions.

Significant amounts of saturated fats and cholesterol are found in whole milk, cheese (especially cream cheese and softer cheeses), cream, butter, ice cream, and sour cream. These fats and cholesterol contribute to cardiovascular diseases, obesity, diabetes, and some forms of cancer. Cow's milk, while high in saturated fat, is also low in the essential fatty acid, linoleic acid. Milk also contains pesticides and drugs. The *New*

England Journal of Medicine (1992) has also reported studies indicating that the vitamin D content of milk samples are mislabeled and are present in potentially toxic amounts.

Menopausal women often ask me if milk is the best source of calcium. They fear that without milk they will have a greater susceptibility to osteoporosis. Neither of these beliefs is true. The highest rates of osteoporosis are in industrialized Western nations where milk is consumed on a daily basis. The incidence of osteoporosis among African-American women, who generally do not consume large quantities of milk, is much less than among Caucasian women. Studies have shown minimal effect of dairy products on osteoporosis. For postmenopausal women, calcium intake has little effect on bone density of the spine or hip. Similarly, calcium intake has relatively little effect on bone density for premenopausal women. Unless a woman is grossly deficient in calcium (consumes less than 400 mg per day), supplements and dairy products have little or no effect. Reducing the risk of osteoporosis depends more on preventing bone loss than on calcium intake.

Increased calcium loss can occur from diets that are high in animal protein. Thus, vegetarians tend to have stronger bones than meat eaters. Caffeine robs the body of calcium. For every six ounces of coffee, five milligrams of calcium are lost through urine, while alcohol inhibits calcium absorption. Smoking also depletes the body of calcium.

One of the most important factors in maintaining healthy bones is exercise. The more the bones are stressed owing to physical activity, the more they hold on to their calcium content.

I teach my patients that good sources of calcium are leafy green vegetables such as kale, turnip greens, collards, Swiss chard, spinach, and escarole. Other foods, such as broccoli, beans, oatmeal, fortified soy milk, and brown rice, are also good sources of calcium. And there are others, such as kelp, dandelion greens, tofu, almonds, and molasses. We need not depend solely on milk.

FIBER

You may have noticed the lack of fresh vegetables and fruits or juices in the above diet diaries. I explain to my patients that the lack of vegetables, whole grains, and fruits is a problem because of a lack of fiber. Why is fiber so important?

We know the lack of dietary fiber has been linked to many diseases associated with Western civilization, such as obesity, diabetes, heart disease, hypertension, and cancer. There are two main types of fiber and both are found in the same food. Soluble fiber—like whole oats, oat bran, chick peas, fruits, and vegetables—is primarily responsible for lowering cholesterol, controlling appetite, and regulating blood sugar. Soluble fiber decreases the time the stomach takes to empty itself and therefore slows down the absorption rate of the food. For both diabetics and nondiabetics this means the normal increase in blood sugar which occurs after a meal is reduced, as are frequent fluctuations in blood sugar. Insoluble fiber, such as the outer shell of brown rice or whole wheat, acts as a natural laxative and increases waste movement through the system.

Fiber has been used for many years in the treatment of constipation. Found in fruits, vegetables, grains, nuts, and seeds, its value is in the fact that it has water-retention properties and thus increases stool size and weight. It is indigestible by humans but its fatty acids are partially degraded by the intestine, producing energy for the intestinal cells. When we eat high-fiber foods such as brown rice and whole-grain breads, the small intestine absorbs the nutrients and the bulky fiber passes into the large intestine. There the fiber absorbs water and is evacuated along with any toxins it has absorbed. An increase of stool weight and size because of increased fiber means a decreased transit time (the time it takes for food to pass from the mouth to the anus).

People in cultures that consume a high-fiber diet (100–170 grams per day) have a transit time of 30 hours and a fecal weight of 500 grams. Americans, on the other hand, who eat a low-fiber diet (20 grams per day) have a transit time of greater than 48 hours and a fecal weight of only 100 grams. Essentially, a larger, bulkier stool passes through the colon more easily, requiring less pressure and force within the colon and therefore less straining. This is one reason a high-fiber diet has been associated with the reduction of cancer, especially colon cancer. A faster transit time allows less time for the colon wall to be exposed to the carcinogens in our waste that result from bacterial degradation of food.

One final word about the general benefits of fiber: foods rich in fiber are called complex carbohydrates (i.e., whole grains, beans, and vegetables) and are known to increase the brain's supply of serotonin, a neurotransmitter that is believed to be responsible for calming and relaxing the mind. And a word of caution about fiber—too much can deplete the body of valuable minerals.

While many Americans are still consuming large amounts of white bread, white sugar, and white rice, the consumption of fiber is not at all foreign to people of color. In fact it is because of Africans that the value of fiber was ever discovered. In the early part of the twentieth century Dr. Price, a dentist, traveled extensively noting orthodontic changes in various cultures that had discontinued their traditional dietary regimes and had begun to eat more Western "civilized" diets. As their diets changed, he noted the beginning of degenerative diseases.

In the 1950s, Dr. Denis Burkitt continued the work of Dr. Price by examining the diets of the people of Kenya and comparing the diseases of those people with those of his country, Britain. He observed that diets low in fiber were associated with high incidences of colon cancer, hiatal hernia, and diverticulosis, ailments that were not common in Africa. Burkitt, along with his colleague, Dr. Hugh Trowell, recorded stages of disease development in third-world cultures. The first stage was based upon the diets of plant eaters who consumed large amounts of fiber. Within these communities there were few examples of degenerative diseases. Obesity and diabetes appeared in the second stage, as diets became more similar to low-fiber diets in the West. The third stage brought with it constipation, hemorrhoids, varicose veins, and appendicitis. With full Westernization of the diet, the fourth stage includes diseases such as ischemic heart disease (decreased blood supply), hypertension, diverticular disease (a protruding or outpouching of the lining of the colon), hiatal hernia, and cancer.

The Detoxification Diet

Because of the value of fiber, I place my patients on a detoxification diet after they have recorded their food intake for five days and returned for their second visit. The detoxification diet is high-fiber—fruits, vegetables, whole grains, nuts, and seeds—low-fat, and lots of fluids in the form of juices (vegetable and fruit) and water, preferably distilled. I ask my patients, with some exceptions, not to eat meat or dairy products during the detox diet. Here is the detoxification diet I give my patients:

DETOXIFICATION DIET

	FOODS TO INCLUDE	FOODS TO AVOID
Beans	Red, pinto, navy, kidney, adsuki, mung, black-eyed peas, chickpeas, split peas, lentils	
Beverages	Herb teas: mint, spearmint, comfrey, red clover, chamomile, licorice, dandelion, chaparral Coffee substitutes: Pero, Cafix, Roma, or Yannoh	Alcohol, cocoa, coffee, milk, soft drinks, decaf coffee
Bread	Millet, rye, buckwheat, whole wheat, bran, corn, 8- or 7-grain, soya tortillas; only whole grains, freshly ground and sprouted, free of all preservatives	White bread and blended bread made with bleached flour
Cereals (Health Valley or New Morning)	Millet, oatmeal, brown and wild rice, buckwheat groats, barley, corn meal, cracked wheat, and 8- or 7-grain. Freshly ground if possible. Quinoa, Amaranth, spelt, kamut	Processed cereals that are puffed, flaked, etc. No white rice
Cheese	None. No dairy products. Tofu (soy cheese) is okay	Forbidden
Dessert	Fresh, whole fruits, fruit cocktails, stewed fruits, natural fruit gelatins, whole tapioca. Sweeten with honey or sorghum to taste. Health desserts made out of ingredients listed	Canned or frozen fruit, all pastries, custards, sauce, ice cream, candy
Eggs	None	Forbidden in any form

Fat	Most cold-pressed unsaturated oils, such as safflower, sesame, walnut, corn, soy, lecithin spread, canola, sunflower, ghee, olive oil (in moderation)	Butter, shortening, margarine, saturated oils and fats, cottonseed oil, rancid and continually heated oils, hydrogenated oils
Fish	None	All fish
Fruits	Fresh fruits, organically grown if possible: apples, apricots, bananas, berries, cherries, currants, grapes, grapefruit, guavas, lemons, mangoes, melons, oranges, papayas, peaches, pears, persimmons, pineapple, plums, tangerines. Use citrus sparingly. Dried fruits, (unsulfured): apples, apricots, dates, figs, peaches, prunes, raisins. Peel sprayed fruits or wash thoroughly	Sprayed and sulfured, canned and frozen
Juices (Knudsen and After the Fall)	Only fresh unsweetened juices if possible. Fruit: apple, berry, cherry, grape, grapefruit, lemon, orange, pear, pineapple, prune. Vegetable: beet, carrot, celery, cucumber, garlic, onion, pepper (red or green bell), radish, red cabbage, turnip. Peel sprayed vegetables or wash thoroughly; dilute all juices with $1/4$ to $1/2$ spring water	All canned frozen juices
Meat	None	All meats in any form
Milk	None. Substitutes: soy (Eden, Vita), sesame, diluted tahini milk,	All dairy and milk products

Rice Dream Milk, oat milk, almond milk. Use nut milks sparingly

Nuts	*Limited amounts* of all kinds of nuts, particularly fresh raw walnuts, almonds, pecans, and peanuts. Raw and nut butters, freshly made in the blender or juicer only	Roasted and salted nuts. Cashews, Brazil, and pine nuts are too high in oils
Potatoes	Baked or steamed with jackets and mashed; potato salad seasoned with salad dressing. Substitute millet, brown rice, and all kinds of noodles and macaroni made from buckwheat, whole wheat, soy, or vegetable flour without eggs	French fries, potato chips, grilled potatoes, white rice, white flour noodles and macaroni
Salads	Use raw fruits and vegetables listed, shredded or chopped, separate and combined, such as shredded apple, carrot, and celery	Sulfur and high-sodium foods
Seasoning	Chives, garlic, parsley, oregano, laurel, basil, marjoram, sage, thyme, and savory. Kelp, vegetable and herb seasonings (that contain no sodium chloride—table salt), and "Vegit" or "Veg Sal" and "Herbamare." Pure apple cider vinegar, sea salt, Dr. Bronner's balanced mineral seasoning, Braggs Liquid Aminos	Spices, black pepper, vinegar
Seeds	Sunflower, chia, sesame, and pumpkin. Fresh and raw	Roasted and salted No seeds such as apple, apricot,

		prunes, plums, peaches, nectarines, cherries, and quince
Soups	Homemade soups made from listed ingredients. Barley, brown rice, or millet can be added	Canned and creamed soup, fat stock, bouillon or dehydrated consommé
Sprouts	Mung, lentil, alfalfa, radish, soy, or wheat (wheat grass manna). Add to salads, sandwiches, or blender drinks	Potato sprouts (poison)
Sweets	Sorghum, raw honey, maple syrup, all in moderation; succanat, stevia, fruit juice, sweetened	White sugar and white sugar products, such as candy and all sugar substitutes
Vegetables, steamed	Raw or freshly cooked, organically grown if possible: artichokes, asparagus, beets, carrots, celery, chives, corn, cucumbers, endive, green and wax beans, green peas, lentils, lima beans, onions, peppers (red and green bell), potatoes, tomatoes, yams, watercress, beet tops, radishes, red cabbage, etc.	Sprayed, canned, and frozen; sulfured and high-sodium foods

*Suggested Menu

Breakfast	Lunch	Dinner
Glass of juice	Salad	Salad
Raw or cooked fruits	Soup	Soup
Cereal with soy milk	Potato	Brown rice or millet,
Soy or rye toast	Cooked vegetables	and tofu, beans,
Multigrain toast		cooked veggies
Tea	Dessert and tea	Fruits and tea

Midmorning	Midafternoon	Evening
Fresh juice or fresh fruit	Fresh juice or fresh fruit	Fresh fruit or unsalted broth

Following the detox diet, I give people a diet for their blood type, which is discussed later in this chapter.

I also ask them to eat as much as possible only foods that are organically grown. This means that the foods they eat will not have been exposed to fertilizers or pesticides as are commercial foods. Why is it necessary to eat organic fruits and vegetables? For the mineral content. Plants don't make minerals and if they don't get them in the soil the plant will not be rich in minerals. Unfortunately, the current methods of farming have depleted the soils, and therefore much of what we eat does not have the mineral nutrition required for good health. The other obvious reason to eat organic foods is so that we do not ingest the pesticide and fertilizer residues in inorganic foods.

But even if we eat whole foods that are organically grown, they will not support our system optimally if we eat too much or eat excesses of one type of food or eat too quickly. So I take the time to give my patients some information on how to create good digestion. Eating excessive amounts of food at one time is a problem simply because the body cannot process it effectively. An excess of meat, dairy, or fatty foods, without vegetables or fruits, will mean that foods pass through the system more slowly. An excess of alcohol or coffee will create a hyperacidic environment which is distressing for the digestive tract. And

*You may desire to eat more frequently on this temporary diet.

eating too quickly, not chewing the food properly, results in decreased digestion because digestion for many foods begins in the mouth.

I also ask that patients do not eat when they are emotionally upset or angry. It is at these times that the sympathetic nervous system is activated. You may know the term "fight or flight." That is the feeling we have when our nervous systems react to the perceived danger or threat. Immediately blood is directed to the extremities and periphery of the body. The result is inhibited digestion. It is when we are relaxed that the parasympathetic nervous system is in control and digestion is made easier.

FOOD COMBINATIONS

Another important aspect of proper digestion also happens to be a fairly controversial topic—proper food combinations. I advise my patients to combine foods properly for many reasons, but primarily because it is healthy. Eating starch (potatoes, rice, bread) with animal protein (meat, poultry, fish) impairs digestion. The enzymes produced by the carbohydrates in the starch and the animal proteins in the meat have difficulty existing together. Thus, digestion is impaired, or at the very least the food takes longer to digest. The microorganisms in the large intestine then have more time to putrefy or ferment the food and create toxins. Imagine if you left food in a garbage pail for several days in the summer. What would happen? The pail would be the host for an abundance of flies, maggots, and perhaps other types of worms and insects. Our intestines are no different if they are filled with undigested foods. While there are microorganisms in our intestines that aid us in making B vitamins, lactic acid, and vitamin K, other microorganisms make over fifty different toxins—ammonia, phenols, indols, alcohol, and formaldehyde, to name several.

Yeast is probably the best-known microorganism of the intestine. The results of overgrowths of this toxin-producing microorganism have been well documented in the books *The Yeast Connection* and *The Yeast Syndrome*. The symptoms can be expressed in many ways. They can be as serious as mental confusion, headaches, dizziness, nausea, and severe, recurrent vaginal yeast infections, or as mild as mild skin irritations or gas and bloating. Antibiotics and refined foods (sugar, white flour, and white rice) have given yeast its popularity and advantage by killing the good bacteria and decreasing digestion, respectively.

Sweet carbohydrates or sugar are of special concern because they are not digested in the mouth or in the stomach but rather in the small intestine. When eaten alone the sugars are sent to the intestines but when eaten with protein or other foods the sugar is held up in the stomach waiting for the other foods to be digested. This produces fermentation of the foods and a haven for yeast.

There are other improper food combinations but suffice it to say, separating starch and animal protein from one another during a meal enables the digestive enzymes of the mouth and stomach to participate more efficiently in the digestive process. More efficient digestion means better elimination of waste and greater absorption of nutrients needed for maximum cellular health.

DRINKING AND EATING

Finally, many people drink water or some other liquid with their meals to ensure they get their eight glasses a day. Drinking with meals is not a good practice. Water and other fluids dilute the digestive juices that are poured into the stomach. When the water passes out of the stomach within ten to fifteen minutes, the digestive juices go along with it and digestion is impeded. Drinking with foods also means that the food is washed down without being properly masticated or chewed. The result is fermentation, putrefaction, and indigestion. I suggest, therefore, that liquids be consumed fifteen to twenty minutes before a meal or fifteen minutes after a meal for maximum digestion.

The purpose of the detoxification diet is to create better elimination through the release of waste or toxins, to allow people to see what they feel like when they eat better, and to begin the process of healing the cells and organs. At the end of the ten-day detoxification, my patients will tell me that they have had more bowel movements in the past ten days than ever before, that their bowels were fuller and easier to pass, and that they have more energy and are sleeping better.

Try this diet for a ten-day period and see how you feel. A word of caution—if you are diabetic or hypoglycemic, have fish four or five times during the ten days. Be sure to have the animal protein with vegetables and salad only to ensure proper food combining.

COLONICS

During and after the ten-day detoxification diet, I suggest that patients receive a series of colonic irrigations. Usually I recommend two or three within a ten- or fifteen-day period, so that some part of the detoxification period overlaps or coincides with the colonics. Subsequently, I suggest patients have up to an additional seven colonics, totaling over ten over a period of six to eight months.

The use of water for therapy (hydrotherapy) is one of the foundations of naturopathic medicine. The colonic is an internal bath that cleanses the colon of toxins such as carbolic acid, indol, and others (see p. 74) named earlier in the chapter. Impacted and putrefied fecal matter is also released during the course of a colonic. When there is old fecal matter in the colon, it is unable to absorb nutrients and eliminate waste properly.

The colon is the end of the digestive process. It is approximately five to six feet long and two and a half inches in diameter. Beginning with the cecum (where it connects to the small intestine), the colon extends up and across the abdominal cavity and down the left side of the body. The sigmoid colon then extends from the descending colon to the rectum and lies in the pelvis. The body uses the colon to absorb minerals, nutrients, and excess water from the digested food we have eaten. It also releases toxins, mucus, gas, and waste from the body. When this process fails, toxins pollute our bodies and dis-ease is the result.

Receiving a colonic is easy and, in most cases, good for you (there are, however, some contraindications—congestive heart failure, active cancer, and swelling of the limbs). To receive a colonic, you lie on a table with your feet toward a colonic machine. This machine has a tank of filtered water, tubing, and levers to turn the water on and off and adjust the water temperature. One end of the tube has a disposable speculum which is inserted gently into the rectum. The machine I use is a gravity machine, which means that the tank is situated above the person on the table. Water flows not by force or control of the colon therapist but by gravity into and out of the rectum through two tubes that are connected to the speculum. As the water flows out of the tube, the colon therapist gently massages your stomach. The machine has a view tube so if you care to you can see the waste leaving your body. The waste goes into a cesspool, as would any waste from a bathroom commode.

Following the detox diet and colonics, patients typically tell me how much lighter and healthier they feel; they have less gas and bloating, easier and more frequent bowel movements, and more energy. Aside from degenerative diseases, fatigue, headaches, and skin problems also are aided by the use of colonics.

As you can imagine, some people are so anxious, depressed, or both that the detoxification diet is too much of a challenge without first reducing some of the anxiety. This is the beauty of being a classical homeopath for me. The homeopathic remedy lifts the mood—replaces the darkness with the light—so that the person is able and willing to make the necessary dietary changes for more healing to occur. The following case will give you an example of what I mean.

A thirty-three-year-old woman came to my office complaining of "stress" and "gastrointestinal problems." Not being fully acquainted with homeopathy, she said she was going to go to someone else to get help with her "breathing problem." She couldn't change her diet because she felt so stressed out. After I asked her about the challenges and issues in her life she told me the following story.

At age seven or nine she had bad tantrums; they were so regular, her parents thought she was epileptic. The doctors prescribed Dilantin and phenobarbital even though they couldn't find anything wrong. The "epilepsy" disappeared until ten years ago, during her last semester in college, when she began to feel anxious about her schoolwork. At the same time, the limbs on the left side of her body felt weak, numb, and heavy.

I noticed she was speaking very quickly and distinctly when she was telling me this. She went to a psychologist who put her on Xanax for three years. Now, seven years later, she suffers from panic attacks during her sleep. They come any time, whether on vacation or during stressful times. After falling asleep at night, she wakes feeling anxious and can't relax enough to calm down and get back to sleep. Sometimes she paces the floor furiously because she has so much energy.

"I can't pace fast enough," she told me. "It must be ninety miles an hour. My left side is trembling and ticking. I have short breath and my heart is racing."

The phenobarbital her doctor suggested doesn't help this jittery insomnia. The next day when she awakens she feels very emotional and cries very easily.

During her childhood, she would get angry if she was teased or hit. Once, during middle school, one of her classmates threw a stone at her on the playground at recess. She warned him not to throw it, but he did it anyway. After school she waited for him outside, tripped him, and hit his head against a brick wall until it bled.

Even during her adolescence she would feel numbness and heaviness in the middle of the night. Her mother would notice that her left side would twist. At age nine, she would black out after experiencing anger and would awaken exhausted. Since the age of twelve or thirteen she had experienced constipation, gas, bloating, and panic attacks on a regular basis.

From a close-knit, middle-class family, she remembered being nasty and aggressive with people who picked on her sister, who let people take advantage of her. As a child, the relationship with her father was quite the opposite, however. One night my patient overheard her parents in a heated argument. She heard loud noises and something falling. When she ran into their room, she found her father forcefully pulling her mother. She yelled out, but he ordered her back to her room and to stay out of their affairs.

"I'm going to kill him," she thought.

This thought was revisited when, as a teenager, her father came into her room and smacked her in the face, knocking her into a door. She ran out of the room to get her father's gun, only to be begged by her mother not to kill her dad. She didn't kill him, nor did she speak to him for three years. But she never stopped wishing he were dead.

The description she gave of her nature was that of someone who liked her privacy and preferred people to think of her as nasty, not nice, so that they would stay away from her. She said she could be nasty, vindictive, and hateful, "a snotty bitch." While giving to people she loves, she can be stubborn and very jealous in relationships. She was, in fact, recently divorced.

As any classical homeopath would do, I questioned her about her fears, sexual behavior, sleep patterns, dreams, food cravings (pasta,

cheese, and bread), and temperature preferences. Her angry and intense nature and subsequent answers confirmed that she needed the
remedy lachesis, made from the venom of the South American bush-
master snake. I gave her lachesis 200 c and asked her to record the
foods that she ate for the next five days. I will tell you more about
lachesis later but first let's look at the diet diary she brought back for
discussion during her second visit.

DAY 1

½ cup bread pudding	7:30 A.M.
½ cup cranberry/grape juice	9:15 A.M.
nutritional drink	9:30 A.M.
6 good and fruity candy	12:00 P.M.
melons, strawberries, grapes	3:00 P.M.
rosemary chicken focaccia	6:00 P.M.
cake	8:00 P.M.
tortilla chips	10:00 P.M.
16 oz. water throughout day	

DAY 2

nutritional drink	8:00 A.M.
banana	11:30 A.M.
coffee	11:35 A.M.
2 slices pizza	9:30 P.M.

DAY 3

nutritional drink	6:30 A.M.
banana	9:30 A.M.
bagel with butter	2:00 P.M.
fish, vegetables, french fries	7:00 P.M.
wine	8:00 P.M.
No bowel movement	

DAY 4

nutritional drink	9:30 A.M.
banana	Noon
grapes and melon	2:00 P.M.
popcorn	2:30 P.M.

hot dog, bagel, chips and salsa	5:30 P.M.
cream-filled cupcakes and ice cream	9:30 P.M.
No bowel movement	

She also reported another condition she omitted during the first interview. She was experiencing dizziness followed by muscular aches. In addition there was one episode of shortness of breath. Her premenstrual mood was noticeably better than it had been before her first visit and generally she thought her mood was better. I felt the remedy was working, but because it had only been two weeks since she had received it I knew I needed to wait until her next visit to see what other effects the remedy would create. She received guidance about the detoxification diet and was asked to return in three weeks.

By her third visit, at the end of six weeks, she reported no muscle pain or shortness of breath and had stopped using inhalers. There was some weakness and numbness of her limbs on the left side but it was markedly reduced. She had not had any panic attacks and was sleeping soundly. She was delighted with the substantial increase in bowel movements and regularity and therefore considerably reduced her use of laxatives. Because her blood group was O, I told her to continue the detoxification diet but to eat animal protein again. I asked her to continue to exclude dairy foods because of her respiratory problems. Over the next four months she became increasingly better, having two minor panic attacks, one of which was related to having problems with an employee. During this time I repeated the homeopathic remedy. The last time I saw this patient, she told me, "I am more in control of myself. I still have some jealousy and can be impatient but I control how I react to situations. My diet is better and I am feeling healthier and stronger. When I eat junk foods I don't feel as well or move my bowels regularly. I can really feel the difference, my system doesn't feel whole as before. I'm just not as well."

This patient clearly responded well mentally and emotionally to the remedy lachesis, as it discontinued her panic attacks. She was now able to have the kind of diet that could make a difference in her physical stamina and well-being.

What do blood group and diet have to do with one another? Everything. Year after year more and more people are becoming vegetarians. As Americans, we are consuming less beef and more chicken and fish.

But should everyone become vegetarian? Should everyone consume animal protein? The answer to both of these questions is "No." To receive maximum benefit from foods, your diet should be based on your blood type.

THE IMPORTANCE OF BLOOD TYPE

By the time I saw Dr. D'Adamo I had been a vegetarian for seven years. I was tired all of the time after the first year of being vegetarian, and while I had had very demanding jobs I thought the fatigue was unusual for a person in her twenties. I thought perhaps I should begin to eat some animal protein, maybe chicken and fish or just fish. It was almost as if my body was telling me to do so. When Dr. D'Adamo told me I should eat some animal protein because my blood type was B, I had never heard of such a thing, but I knew instinctively he was right. He was not advocating dieting but rather eating well and allowing the nutrients to support my body while the toxins—waste and water—were being released in the process.

As a result of my personal experience and now ten years of professional practice, I have witnessed vegetarians renew their health and vitality by eating animal protein. And I have watched meat eaters find tremendous relief from allergies, asthma, and arthritis by becoming vegetarian.

Naturopaths believed that most people should be vegetarians. This was especially necessary for any healing to take place. Dr. D'Adamo explained to me on one of my visits that he thought, if we are all different people, how could it be that we all need to eat the same foods? He believed there had to be a way to discern more definitively what foods people should eat. During his days at the Kneipp Institute he was impressed by the healing response to a vegetarian diet and hydrotherapy (water therapy in the form of colonics, baths, and showers). But he became aware that some patients may have cured their illnesses but were listless, pale, weak, and depressed after being vegetarian for six or eight months. Some were so fatigued, they felt disconnected from their everyday affairs. Others had severe muscle atrophy.

It was in Germany in the 1960s during further study that he learned why some foods are more suitable than others, depending on the individual. Doctors there spoke frequently of how German doctors during World War II tried to develop diets for soldiers for maximum nutrition. Now his colleagues were questioning if blood type could determine what a person should eat. Dr. D'Adamo knew that blood was the life force of our bodies in that it carries oxygen, controls body temperature, determines immunity against diseases, and circulates nutrients. He decided to use blood groups to determine what nutrients the body needs. What he found was something truly groundbreaking.

WHAT ARE BLOOD GROUPS?

Antigens, one of the components of our immune system, are found on the surface of our red blood cells. Their purpose is to detect any foreign invaders in the body and decide whether they are harmful or beneficial. When a harmful pathogen enters your body, your antigens produce antibodies which attach themselves to the foreign substance so they can be disposed of easily through the body's eliminatory processes.

Your blood type is determined by the type of antigen that exists on your cells. If you have an A antigen, then your blood type or group is A. If you have a B antigen on your cells, then your blood type is B. If you have both A and B antigens on your cells, however, your blood type is AB (universal receiver). And if you have no antigens on your red blood cells your blood group is O (universal donor). Blood groups were discovered in 1900 by Dr. Karl Landsteiner, for which he received a Nobel Prize in 1930, when he realized that blood groups produced antigens to other blood groups. Dr. Landsteiner discovered that group A carried anti-B antibodies, and blood group B carried anti-A antibodies. This meant that people with these two blood types cannot exchange blood because if they did the blood would clump together. Blood group AB had no antibodies, making it the only blood group to be able to receive anyone's blood, and blood group O carried both anti-A and anti-B antibodies. Thus, O can receive only O blood but can donate blood to anyone (A or B or AB).

DIETS AND BLOOD GROUPS: A HISTORY

When Dr. D'Adamo opened his own practice in the 1950s he began to obtain the blood groups of all of his patients and observe their responses to diets. He discovered that people with blood type A have a very difficult time assimilating dairy products and animal protein. These foods produced more mucus in type A people. Essentially, they could obtain all of their nutrients from a vegetarian diet barring any severe pathology. People with blood type O were the exact opposite. They required animal protein and over time became weakened by a vegetarian diet. Foods best suited for blood type B and AB were combinations and moderations of the A and O diets.

He also recognized that blood group O people were people who needed exercise and physical activity. Their bodies were heavy, unlike the blood group A people, whose bodies tended to be more slender and fragile. B blood type presented physiques that were somewhere in the middle, not very muscular or fragile.

In 1980, Dr. D'Adamo wrote a book, *One Man's Food Is Someone Else's Poison,* which explains his theories and observations regarding the optimal diets for various blood types. As I read this book I wondered about the exact connection between diet and blood type. I wondered if this mystery, like so many, had its roots in Africa, the "Cradle of Civilization."

I remember in the 1960s, along with consciousness of Dr. Martin Luther King, Jr., and President John F. Kennedy, there was the awareness "Black Is Beautiful." African-Americans were finally learning and taking pride in the fact that Africa was the "Cradle of Civilization" and not the "Dark Continent" full of monkeys and cannibals. As a freshman and sophomore in college my minor was anthropology. In my anthropology classes in the 1960s and during the writing of my dissertation in the 1970s I recall learning and writing about the origin of our "Negroid" features of thick lips, kinky hair, and large nostrils—adaptations to the geographical location of Africa. As we migrated to less temperate climates humans lost the need for those attributes and had fairer skin to protect against the cold and absorb more vitamin D, straighter hair, and less massive facial structures. As we changed and migrated, so did our blood groups and nutritional requirements. Any story of the beginning of time starts in Africa and travels to other continents and countries. The story of human beings and their diets is no different.

Recently, Dr. D'Adamo's son, Peter J. D'Adamo, N.D., used this knowledge to explain the link between diets and blood groups in his book *Eat Right 4 Your Type* (1996). Subsequent to the age of the Neanderthals, Cro-Magnon men became the most dangerous predators (40,000 B.C.) on the planet. They hunted in packs and ultimately made

weapons for the purpose of killing their prey. Their strength and physical abilities were superior. Everyone was blood type O and their diet
was meat-based. As the population expanded, so did the need for animal protein. Humans started fighting one another for food and territory
where food could be hunted. The competition was so great that migration was the only option. By 30,000 B.C. hunters were traveling farther
to find meat. With topographical and climatic changes, they migrated
out of Africa to Europe and Asia; thus, the reason for the preponder-
ance of blood group O on the planet. Around 20,000 B.C., Cro-Mag-
nons had killed much of the animal life in Europe and Asia so that other
foods had to be found. At that point they began to feed on both plants
and animals—eating berries, shrubs, roots, and small animals. The
larger the population, the more need for food and the more need to
fight for it. Migration continued.

As a result of the migration from Africa and subsequent dietary and
environmental adaptations there was a change in the digestive tracts
and immune systems of people. This change created the blood group A
in Asia or the Middle East between 25,000 and 15,000 B.C. These people cultivated grains and livestock and were therefore able to establish
communities and have a more permanent lifestyle. With new agricultural demands, they needed to plan for the future and cooperate with
one another. Organizational skills such as problem solving and coordi-
nating tasks were necessary for this population, not hunting. As with
any mutation, the people lived longer and healthier and, most importantly for evolution, had more children. They survived the infections of
heavily populated areas in greater numbers than blood group O. Eventually moving into western Europe and parts of Russia and creating
peoples of Iran and Afghanistan, different diets were introduced into
the digestive tracts of the hunters. The hunters lost their ability to survive solely on animal protein.

Between 10,000 and 15,000 B.C. blood type B appeared among
Caucasian and Mongolian tribes in what are now Pakistan and India.
Two different B groups moved into Asia, one agrarian and sedentary,
the other nomadic and warlike. The nomads moved into eastern Europe
and those dependent upon agriculture migrated throughout China and
southeast Asia. They developed very sophisticated irrigation techniques
that exemplify their creativity and intelligence. When the A blood type
of Caucasians mixed with the B blood type of Mongolians the result

was blood type AB. It is the most recent and the least common of all the blood types.

BLOOD TYPE O

The lachesis patient is an example of blood type O. Recall she was pacing, aggressive, hateful, vindictive, and jealous. That is not to say all blood type O's have this personality. Quite the contrary. They can have the complete opposite personality, but I've noted those in my practice all have in common a certain hardiness and strength. They are goal-oriented, directed and focused, but not necessarily creative. While not as energetic as blood type A's, they do require strenuous physical exercise to stimulate them mentally, emotionally, and physically. Exercise is imperative. It releases tension, increases their ability to concentrate, memorize, and be creative. Their digestive processes depend upon exercise as well. The colon is, after all, a muscle.

I tell type O patients if they have an exam to study for, exercise for one hour and then study for an hour. While many of them don't particularly like to exercise, they feel much better afterward. They appear muscular and solid.

Though fiber and other foods on the detoxification diet are essential for everyone, meat (lean veal, lamb, chicken, turkey) is an equally essential part of the O diet. Like their ancestors, O's generally need a high-energy food—the protein complement that is found in animals. Typically 3–6 ounces of meat three times a week and 4–6 ounces of poultry two times a week are sufficient. Specific fish are also important: bluefish, cod, halibut, herring, mackerel, rainbow trout, red snapper, salmon, sardine, sole, and striped bass. I usually recommend 4–6 ounces, two times a week. Notice I do not recommend shellfish because they are high in cholesterol and inhabit the bottom of the ocean, eating the debris of the other fish.

Type O's can digest meat more efficiently because of the high amounts of hydrochloric acid in the stomach. (This is one reason why blood type O's who are vegetarian may have a high rate of ulcerative conditions because there is no animal protein in the diet to digest.) This is another reason why exercise is so important: because it releases toxins, like uric acid, that can build up from meat and cause kidney problems and arthritis, for example.

Type O individuals have a very wide range of foods to eat, but they do not tolerate dairy products well. Remember that most African-Americans and most other people are lactose-intolerant. Whole wheat products also are not particularly good for blood type O. They do better with grains like those listed on the detoxification diet, such as kamut, spelt, quinoa, and millet.

Vegetables for blood group O should include collards, kale, dandelion greens, escarole, beet greens, okra, broccoli, pumpkin, parsnips, red peppers, spinach, Swiss chard, and sweet potatoes.

BLOOD GROUP A

The complete opposite of O, blood group A *must* be vegetarian (there are exceptions as mentioned, such as diabetics and hypoglycemics). I tell patients that this doesn't have to happen overnight. But within a year's time they should be vegetarian—gradually removing red meat, then chicken, and finally fish from their diet. Meat and dairy products always constipate and congest a person with blood group A. Because type A's have low acid content in the stomach, digesting meats is very difficult. Dairy is not only hard to digest but provokes insulin reactions and is high in saturated fat. Wheat is a poor choice of food for this blood group as well, since it creates too much acid in the muscles.

One patient who came into the office told me he was eating chicken and turkey again and noticed that his bowels were not moving as well. He was sluggish and his stool was hard. This did not surprise me, based on the fact that he was blood type A. "I'm back to being vegetarian now and things are fine," he told me later after following my advice to avoid meats.

For those who have a particularly hard time being vegetarian, I will recommend some fish like cod, grouper, mackerel, red snapper, rainbow trout, salmon, and sardine. They may be able to have a bit of yogurt and 2 percent cottage cheese. But most of their protein should come from soy cheese and soy milk, tofu, and beans. Aduke, adzuki, pinto, lentils, black-eyed peas are especially beneficial. Grains should be sprouted if they are wheat (the gluten which can be a problem for A's is destroyed in the sprouting process). Rice and soy flours are recommended as well as millet, spelt, oat bran, buckwheat, and rye crisps.

Vegetables that are a necessary part of the diet are: artichokes, beet leaves, broccoli, carrots, collard greens, dandelion greens, escarole, kale, okra, onions, parsnips, spinach, and Swiss chard. Avoid cabbage as it can be gaseous for A's, and tomatoes because they can agglutinate (clump) the blood.

Fruits like oranges and bananas should be avoided by blood group A. Oranges irritate the alkaline stomach of the A and bananas are hard to digest. Especially good for blood group A's are berries, figs, grapefruit, pineapple, plums, prunes, and raisins.

In my practice I observe type A's to be of very high intelligence and possess very analytical minds. They always have a thought or plan or project—so many that to accomplish them all is a problem. Blood group A's are busy. They have nervous energy and find exercise necessary to release nervous tension but their mental energy suffers as a result. They are more mental than physical and need to relax the mind and nervous system with disciplines like yoga, tai chi, and meditation. They tend to be disciplined, organized, orderly, bordering on fastidious and anxious. Worry is a big part of their lives. They can be pessimistic and inflexible.

BLOOD GROUP B

Blood group B combines the best of both worlds—the high intellect and empathy of the blood group A, as well as the physical aggression of the blood group O. B's are moderators, or counselors, the ones who create order out of chaos and the ones to whom people will come and share their problems. They are both practical and creative with an intuitive understanding of what does and does not work in the world. They are motivators of people and good communicators. I have observed that they are flexible, independent, direct, persuasive, and sensitive.

Moderation is the key for blood group B's. They need to be vegetarian several days a week and eat animal protein two or three days a week. The dietary requirements resemble both A and O. They react to whole wheat like blood group O's, and should avoid it. Other foods that are problematic are corn, peanuts, and buckwheat, all of which cause blood sugar problems. Unfortunately, chicken is a food that many blood group B's do not assimilate well. This is due to the fact that there is a type B agglutinating (clumping) factor in the muscle tissue of the chicken. I suggest they eat other poultry and fish, not chicken. Fish is the mainstay of blood group B's, especially salmon, halibut, whitefish, sole and flounder, grouper, and sardine. Again I urge you to avoid shellfish.

Dr. Peter D'Adamo says that blood type B's can tolerate dairy foods because they were introduced to the diet at the height of blood type B development. I don't find that to be the case in my practice. Most of my African-American patients seem to be lactose-intolerant and my Caucasian patients seem to have allergies to dairy foods. Perhaps the allergies are due to the region where I live—Washington, D.C., is in a valley and allergies are abundant.

Most vegetables are beneficial for blood group B's, but from my professional experience, I believe tomatoes and corn should be eliminated from the diet. Vegetables that should be consumed are beets, broccoli, cabbage, carrots, collards, kale, lima beans, mustard greens, red peppers, yellow peppers, and sweet potatoes.

Moderation in exercise is also important—hiking, cycling, tennis, jogging, and swimming are all beneficial for the blood group B's, but do not need to be practiced daily as with a blood group O. Two or three times per week is sufficient. To maintain mental/emotional balance, I tell patients to include yoga, tai chi, and/or meditation as well.

BLOOD TYPE AB

People of this blood group should be vegetarians who have a little bit of fish and chicken in their diet. After all, they are both A and B. They are sensitive and high-strung like an A, yet balanced and diplomatic like a B. They are honest, organized, and have a strong intuition. They can be easily offended and sentimental. Cycling and swimming are preferred for blood group AB, not the strenuous sports of tennis or jogging. Most importantly, they need the calming of yoga and the movement that tai chi provides. Deep breathing and relaxation are essential for good health as the immune system of the AB can be made very susceptible to disease through stress.

People who are type AB should eat lamb, turkey, and fish, especially cod, grouper, mackerel, monkfish, rainbow trout, red snapper, salmon, and sardine. Tofu should be a regular part of the diet for added protein. Dairy in the form of egg whites and yogurt work best for the digestion of AB.

Grains like millet, brown rice, soy flour, sprouted wheat, oat bran, oatmeal, rice bran, and spelt are best for this blood group. And vegetables are similar to A and B blood group requirements: beet leaves, beets, broccoli, celery, collard greens, cucumber, dandelion greens, eggplant, kale, mustard greens, parsnips, sweet potatoes, and alfalfa sprouts.

Fruits like grapes, grapefruit, kiwi, lemons, pineapples, and plums are good sources of vitamins and minerals for type AB's.

Regardless of blood type, I ask every patient to begin the morning with the juice of ¼ to ½ lemon in 6 to 8 ounces of bottled water in order to cleanse the system of mucus and stimulate the bowel. For blood types A and AB, I suggest warm water. For blood types O and B, I recommend room-temperature water.

BLOOD GROUPS O, A, B, AB—ONE RACE

Facts about migration and blood grouping have been written about for many years by anthropologists and biologists. For ten years my practice has borne witness to the concept that blood type determines nutritional needs. This observation, as well as theories about personality traits, extend beyond "racial" characteristics. Often we have more in common with someone who shares our blood group than with someone within our "race."

Though racism is the most chronic and serious disease in America, there are no grounds for it. Racism is for the purpose of supporting misunderstandings and preconceived ideas about people and discriminatory practices against those people. There are no anthropological reasons to classify people into races. People in India are classified as "Caucasoid" yet many have darker skin than "black" Americans. Likewise, many "Negroid" people in sub-Saharan Africa have skin lighter than or as dark as many people in Mediterranean countries. And there are people in New Guinea who are black, with woolly hair, who have no ancestral ties to Africa. We are one race, one people—division by "race" is man's will, not God's will.

Eat well, live long, love one another . . .

PART TWO

THE PATH
CONTINUES

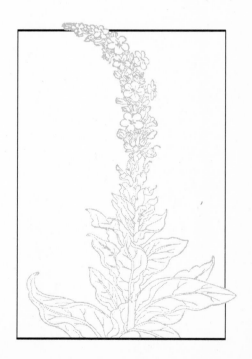

A NOTE

During my sophomore year of college I read the Kerner Commission Report for a class I took on race relations. The Kerner Commission Report, as most people can remember, was released in 1968 in response to the race riots of that year. Among the findings of this commission was the following statement:

> America is, and has always been, a racist society. Bigotry penetrates every level and every region of the country, North and South, business, labor, journalism, education and medicine. The causes [of racism] are ignorance, apathy, poverty and above all a pervasive discrimination that has thwarted each and every American Negro in all avenues of his life.

The report continued by saying racism was the cause of the disunion and division in American life. Although the report is nearly thirty years old, its conclusion is still truthful to this day, and the damaging consequences linger with us now.

The Kerner Report isn't the only official finding that speaks to these problems. An article in the *Journal of Black Psychology* (1996) states that, regardless of class, African-Americans report racist events so often that depression, rage, and tension about racism are the most common problems among African-Americans in psychotherapy. Not surprisingly, the study found that stress-related symptoms such as depression, anxiety, insecurity, as well as physical symptoms like headaches and backaches, were significantly associated with the frequency of racist events. It is worth noting that the National Institutes of Health, one of the most respected medical institutions in the world, agreed with these findings, saying that racism "undoubtedly had negative consequences for our physical and mental health."

This discrimination is found at all levels of society. African-Americans experience it when looking for a new house or apartment, or when applying for a job or a loan. But more than anything else we experience it on the most obvious level: face-to-face interaction with strangers. Whether falsely accused of stealing or cheating, given poor service in restaurants and stores, or simply avoided like pariahs on the street, we never forget the personal encounters with this common form of hatred.

I am sure many African-Americans can remember an act of discrimination that in some way affected our health, but let me give you a personal example. My office is located in a high-rent area of Washington, D.C. It has a history of being predominantly white, though that has slowly been changing in recent years. On the way home from work one day last year, I was about three blocks from my office when a car quickly crossed over into my lane in front of me. I heard a loud noise that sounded as if something hit my car. The driver of the car in front obviously heard it, too, because he pulled over and jumped out to investigate. I pulled over too.

I saw a hubcap near our cars and immediately realized it had careened off another car and rolled into our paths. This man, however, obviously did not see it.

"What the hell is wrong with you, nigger bitch?" he yelled out.

"Excuse me?" I replied in a tone of disbelief and confusion.

He was Caucasian, well dressed, and appeared, to all intents and purposes, to be intelligent. "How could such a circumstance create such a vile reaction?" I thought. I told him I felt sorry for him because he was so ignorant, and got back in my car.

I have had enough experience over the years to handle this type of situation, but nevertheless I was flustered. How dare he say that to me? He can say that because he is dis-eased from the hatred and fear of a people because of color. These racist situations are demeaning and personal because they attack an essential fact of being African-American. Nothing else compares to this type of stress. No exam, no late appointment, no work deadline creates as much short-term and long-term stress as a situation like the one I had with this hateful driver.

As if this were not enough, we are also victims of the American sick care system, a system that focuses on disease and on maintaining the body, no matter the quality of life. Racism aside, the current medical system overlooks wellness and prevention. Costs for traditional health care have escalated because patients have learned to go to doctors frequently, often inappropriately, to get a "quick fix" of expensive prescription drugs.

State and federal subsidies for medical students also account for high costs in health care. As subsidies increase, so do the number of graduating medical students. This would not be a problem if many of these graduates became general practitioners. But they do not. Instead, most graduates, lured by the promise of making hundreds of thousands a year, opt to enter a specialty field, where they can charge more for services and order the most expensive and at times unnecessary procedures and prescriptions.

In the past ten years the number and cost of prescriptions have increased from an average of $5.50 for one drug per person, per year, to *six and one half drugs per person, per year, with an average cost of $22.50 per drug.* Drug companies claim the higher prices are due to increased costs of research and development, but in reality drug companies spend three times more money on advertising than on research. Since 1950 the drug industry has been the most profitable business in America.

The overuse of drugs has caused more problems. Recent research tells us that preventable, drug-related diseases and deaths cost $77 billion a year. The elderly are especially vulnerable and suffer greatly from the misuse of drugs. Being on an average of thirteen drugs each year, they take 40 percent of all prescription drugs, resulting in a 10 percent incidence of adverse conditions.

Even with all of the technology, drugs, and surgeries, our health as a nation has not improved. We may live longer but not in healthy, productive ways. The improvements in health over the century are not due to drugs and surgery but rather to successful public health programs that reduced bacteria in our water and food supplies, thereby preventing infectious diseases.

We owe something to ourselves, our ancestors and our children—to increase the quality of our own lives. It is time to stop waiting for an end-stage disease to strike and then taking that body part to a specialist. As I said in an earlier chapter, health has to be accomplished by working in concert with your body's wisdom and a health care practitioner who respects that wisdom. As a team, you can concentrate on primary prevention of disease. If there are signs from the body that something is not right, and that assistance is necessary, then that too can be accomplished. If these efforts fail, drugs and surgery will always be available.

The Deadliest Diseases

Based on what I have seen in my practice, the "deadliest diseases" covered in the second part of this book affect a majority of our nation but are the most common and most damaging ailments that plague black America. It is critical that we African-Americans not only recognize these diseases but confront them with preventive care. These short, instructional chapters are intended to be used in conjunction with the more general information outlined in Part One of this book. Natural medicine is complementary medicine, not alternative medicine. It does not conflict with conventional medicine.

As you read the following chapters, please be aware that any of the conditions discussed may require a different homeopathic remedy for each individual being treated. The diets and herbal preparations may be more generic and may be applied in more general terms without complications. Anyone treating himself for periods of six months or more without improvement and/or anyone who is somehow adversely affected by a homeopathic medicine or an herbal regimen needs to seek the advice of a naturopathic physician.

5

STRESS

Like most doctors, I have my patients fill out a questionnaire on their first visit. I ask the usual questions. Are they on any medications or medical treatments? Are they suffering from any diseases or ailments? Do they have any allergies? Their responses vary widely on almost all of the questions except one: Why have they come to my office? Approximately half of all of my patients answer "Stress." But among my African-American patients, 60 to 70 percent of the responses are stress along with other conditions, like hypertension, diabetes or arthritis, diseases which are disproportionately prevalent among blacks.

WHAT IS STRESS?

Stress strains the body. It can be physical, mental or emotional in form, but it is always a specific response to some stimulus, such as pain or fear, that disrupts a person's normal body function. When stress is evident, the sympathetic nervous system responds by what you may have heard of as "fight or flight." When we cannot respond in those ways, however, and we have to suppress our instincts in order to conform, we have continual stress. We can have hormonal imbalances—like increased adrenal hormones—that play an important role in regulating blood pressure, for example. The imbalance of the adrenal hormone also interferes with blood sugar utilization and insulin sensitivity, as is the case with diabetics.

Another part of the nervous system, such as the parasympathetic nervous system, is depressed during stress. This system is responsible for bodily functions when the body is at rest or asleep. Under stress these systems are out of balance.

Stress also suppresses immune function—the system that is responsible for destroying foreign microorganisms and generally maintaining our health. White blood cell function and production are inhibited when we are under stress. White blood cells perform a variety of functions, primarily to make antibodies and respond to foreign substances in the body, like bacteria and viruses.

Hans Selye at the University of Prague in the 1920s is the person whom we credit for the early work done on stress and illness. And subsequent research has told us that emotional stress can cause a susceptibility to disease. This is the understanding we have had for years, decades in naturopathy and homeopathy.

Years after Selye's initial work, a scale was developed at the University of Washington School of Medicine that speaks to the type of stress—separation, divorce, imprisonment, death of a partner, etc.—that can create physical problems. Each stressful occurrence has attached to it a numerical value. Depending on how high one scores on the scale will determine the likelihood of getting a disease. It does not speak to how an individual responds to stress, however.

The level of stress we experience depends on the amount of stimuli and how we respond to them. The same stress is handled differently by different people. And people have developed and participate in different techniques to handle their stress—exercise, meditation, vacations, yoga, etc. So stress can be caused by something minor, like speaking in public, or something profound, like the death of a loved one. In either instance, stress makes people more susceptible to spiritual, mental, emotional, and physical dis-ease. And to be susceptible means to be more accessible to harmful disease.

One's susceptibility to disease changes as situations and circumstances change. Through the relatively new discipline of psychoneuroimmunology (the study of how the mind and emotions affect the nervous and immune systems), mainstream medicine has finally acknowledged that there is a relationship between mind and body and that they may have a significant effect on each other.

Stress is undeniably one of the most dangerous problems affecting the health of all Americans today. And it is as closely tied to African-

Americans as the color of our skin. Stress will impact African-Americans at every level of identity, as individuals, or as members of a group, or on an affiliation level, for example, not being allowed to join a certain country club or reside in a certain neighborhood.

Caucasian Americans do not have the same type of stress at the affiliation, group, or individual level of identity. Because of American history and sheer numbers, the stress of Caucasians is different, though damaging nonetheless. We cannot change history and its consequences. People of color are obvious. Caucasians of all ethnicities melt into the fabric and pattern of America. But I have come to understand that, while our stresses may be different and everyone responds to stress differently, feelings of low self-esteem, isolation, and depression are rampant in this society, among all people.

I recall a young Caucasian woman who came to me very "stressed out," complaining of repeated upper respiratory problems and vaginal infections. After spending time with her I learned that she had a young child who was very active and defiant and that she had recently married a man who was not the baby's father. The father of the child left her while she was pregnant. She had known her current husband two months before they began to live together; they planned to marry in the next six months but he backed out of that agreement and she had to cancel all of the wedding plans. They then resumed the relationship and had recently married.

She had had abortions in the past and could not allow herself to terminate a pregnancy again. Now that she was married and had a child she felt trapped, alone, overwhelmed and unsupported. But these feelings began in childhood.

"My mom was never there for me. I have had three fathers, and I was not close to any of them. I never knew my real dad. I found out where he lived and called him and he would not talk to me. I called my uncle to ask him if he could make my father talk to me. He said that my father said he could not talk to me. He never paid child support, so Mom got married to try to make things right. For my mom it was always men first, money second, and then me." She continued by saying she always felt alone, and as if she was in her mother's way. Once her mother asked Joan if she liked the man she was about to marry. Even though Joan said no her mother married him anyway, telling Joan she would just have to deal with the marriage. Joan dealt with it through the use of drugs and alcohol beginning at age fourteen.

One of her mother's husbands was an alcoholic who physically abused her mother. He would also come into Joan's room at night, drunk and naked, and sit on the side of the bed and talk to her. Though he did not overtly abuse her, Joan was scared and confused. "I have been desperately seeking stability. I never got to be a child and feel safe as a child should feel. I felt alone a lot. I have not developed skills of an adult because no one took time with me. I do not feel good about myself."

As I said in the Introduction, I agree with Francis Hargrave: we have all suffered from the institution of slavery. As a people, one people, our morals or standards with respect to right and wrong behavior have been reduced to a goal. Our passions—emotions and sexual desire/lust—dominate our reason and ethical principles. Just as African slaves taught their offspring, so the Caucasian masters taught theirs.

I am aware that some of this unrestrained passion has also been let loose upon Caucasian women as I hear the countless stories of incest victims. Ultimately feeling powerless, angry, fearful, and worthless, all victims of incest suffer a range of problems, from severe debilitating depression and anxiety to severe premenstrual symptoms or chronic bladder and yeast infections. From a very young age through age fifteen, Susan was victimized by her grandfather and then her father. "I am afraid people will hurt me. I do not want to be out with a lot of people. If they want something from me and I cannot deliver, I believe something bad may happen to me, so I do not want to be close to too many people. Sometimes it's like I don't want them to know me because I am so bad. If they get to know me they will figure out that I am not a good person. If they know my desires and preferences I will be laughed at and ridiculed. I will be annihilated. I feel unsafe and terrified if I don't fit in; like a target, an impaled animal. I have dreams of women trying to kill me and I couldn't get them to stop looking at me."

Susan's mother was of no support as she dominated Susan as well, but in a different way. She was overprotective, making all of Susan's decisions for her, never allowing for Susan's opinions and desires. Yet she seemed oblivious to what was happening between her daughter and her husband. "I couldn't exist as myself beside her. I couldn't be apart from her either because she wouldn't let me. I felt buried by her. I always had to be a good daughter. I am afraid of being angry. When I allow myself to get angry I get happier, I feel powerful. I will hit the chair until my knuckles bleed."

Severe migraine headaches were the reason Sandra, who is also Caucasian, came to my office. But after visiting with her for an hour and a half, I heard a story of mental and emotional abuse, and finally sexual molestation. "I grew up thinking I was fat, dumb, and ugly. I tried to be perfect, but nothing was good enough for my parents, especially my dad. I was never allowed to have my own mind or thoughts about anything. I always felt like I had to do what they said or something bad would happen. Nobody would like me because I was a bad person, and my parents wouldn't love me. My father would blow up at me and yell and scream. I never felt good enough or smart enough."

After telling me more details about her family, she revealed a dark secret that had been with her for many years. "There is something else I need to tell you about that is hard to talk about," she said. "I was molested by a friend of the family. I never told anyone then because he said if I did, he would kill me. I think it may be one of the reasons I have migraine headaches—because of all the pressure."

Naturopathic and homeopathic physicians have known that our susceptibility to disease is directly related to our emotional condition, whether we are grieving, angry, anxious, or fearful, and to our physical condition. The extent of one's susceptibility to disease is directly related to situations and circumstances that decrease immune defenses such as grief, anger, anxiety, and fear. And so it is with physical influences like poor nutrition, inadequate or excessive exercise, inadequate sleep or insomnia and little or no recreation. Both physical and emotional conditions influence susceptibility to disease.

A SPECIAL NOTE: While stress affects every segment of our population, the following 12 pages speak specifically to stress as it affects blacks in America, because I believe there is an added dimension to stress for people of color. That added dimension is racism, whether it be covert or overt. Although my compassion runs deep for all, I understand best, by experience, the stress of people of color. I cannot in good conscience exclude information that I know is directly relevant to this topic of stress, and what I believe is essential for healing to take place.

If you are not a person of color, it is my sincere desire that you too read this section and that it may enlighten you as you continue on your path to healing.

BEING BLACK IN AMERICA AS A
SOURCE OF STRESS

OUR PAST AS SLAVES

Slavery created constant, obvious, immediate, and certain stress. These Africans, whose psyches were crippled, were responsible, through the generations, for our self-identity and socialization, our integrity and self-esteem.

Slavery will always be a terrible scar in American history. Its legacy of pain and fear still resonates within the African-American community today. At least once a month for the past ten years I have heard a story of racism and discrimination from a patient. It may be as simple as being called a racial epithet or it may be as complicated as being passed over for a promotion for ambiguous reasons. In some ways, the hand of racism is more threatening today because it is no longer as visible. When a sales clerk shadows an African-American around a store to make sure he isn't shoplifting, how many shoppers notice? The African-American surely does. He feels the mistrust and the stress of being targeted in the store based purely on his physical profile.

In November 1995 this unseen practice attracted national attention in an incident near Washington, D.C., when a white security guard at an Eddie Bauer store forced an African-American teenager to literally take the shirt off his back. The guard thought it had been shoplifted, even though the young man had purchased the shirt the day before. The guard and another white coworker made him leave the shirt at the register.

The story made national news and provoked outrage at the Eddie Bauer company. For African-Americans who have experienced similar forms of abuse, it reaffirmed the racism that is prevalent in retail stores. But more importantly, it permanently damaged the faith and hope of this law-abiding black man, who was humiliated in front of his friend, in front of a large crowd of Christmas shoppers, and in front of the staff at the store.

In August 1997, New York City police officers, after arresting a young Haitian man for his alleged involvement in a disturbance outside a nightclub, shouted racial epithets, brutally beat and sodomized him while in police custody at Brooklyn's 70th Precinct. The charges against the man were immediately dropped.

Incidents like this remind us that racism still lingers. Anyone who believes the effects of slavery are long past need only review the history of slavery in America. The first colony, Jamestown, was settled in 1607. The first African slaves were brought to this continent in 1620, more than *a hundred and fifty years* before this land became a country. And even though slavery was abolished at the end of the Civil War in 1865, Jim Crow laws and racial discrimination lingered for another hundred years, until civil rights laws, passed in the fifties and sixties, made racial discrimination illegal. When viewed from this broader perspective, it is easier to see the long, uphill battle African-Americans face. Thirty years of reparations cannot make up for more than three hundred and fifty years of slavery and oppression.

My hundred-and-one-year-old grandmother told me she knew very little of her grandmother, a slave. My grandmother's mother never spoke about much, especially of her mother. It was too painful. And my grandfather told me of his horror and pain as he watched the Ku Klux Klan kill his grandfather. It was a hate crime, plain and simple, driven by fear. Just as I am the descendant of a slave, so too is someone out there the descendant of a Ku Klux Klan member. As my grandparents spoke, I felt their pain. I became angry and wondered how different their lives could have been without the shackles of racism. This anger and hurt caused stress. Many of my patients have other memories with similar reactions. The past and present are closely bound together.

THE STRESS OF EMANCIPATION

Africans and their offspring helped build this country with their lives. We have a deep investment in America. We took better care of our masters' children than our own, and we continue to do so as nannies and live-in caregivers. We nursed the sick and dying, both black and white. We have taken care of everyone but ourselves.

Black women especially have had to care for children, parents, lovers, spouses, and parents of spouses. As Opal Palmer Adisa says in *Body and Soul: The Black Women's Guide to Physical Health and Emotional Well-Being*:

> Did you ever wonder why sisters look so angry? Why we walk like we've got bricks in our bags and will slash and curse you at the drop of a hat? It's because stress is hemmed into our dresses, pressed into our hair, mixed in our perfume, and painted on our fingers. *Stress* from the deferred dreams, the dreams not voiced; *stress* from always being at the bottom, from never being thought of as beautiful; *stress* from being a Black woman in America. . . . [Emphasis mine.]

Black women have been and still are the domestic support for the nation, while our lives—our very selves—have been negated and neglected. And so the stress continues.

And what about African-American men? Black men rank at the bottom in nearly every survey and measurement related to quality of life, but at the same time rank near the top in categories like imprisonment, disease, and early death. According to the U.S. Department of Justice, roughly one third of all African-American men in their twenties are in prison, on parole, or otherwise connected to the criminal justice system, while only one in fifteen white men in the same age group is in a similar situation. Only one black man goes to college for every one hundred who go to jail. African-Americans are at least twice as likely to be unemployed as whites, and more than half of all African-American men between the ages of twenty-five and thirty-four are either not employed or do not earn enough to support a family of four above the poverty level.

As a group blacks are negated, neglected, disrespected, ridiculed, and denigrated. When I worked at the Department of Housing and Urban Development, my colleagues and I often had conversations about public housing issues. I was troubled to hear my white coworkers refer to black people as if we were another species, without feelings, rights, or thoughts. I was too embarrassed, hurt, and angry to say anything.

I recall having lunch one day with several of my white colleagues. The restaurant we went to served upscale American cuisine. Its tables were covered with immaculate white linen and its wait staff wore starched white shirts and silk ties. Having come to this restaurant on many other occasions, I casually noticed that fewer African-American men were waiting tables, and how, in this restaurant and others, Hispanic men had taken their place as waiters and bus boys.

"Well, maybe it's because Hispanics are better workers," one colleague said.

I looked around the table. A few others nodded in assent.

"What exactly do you mean by that?" I said.

"What I mean," this man across from me explained, "is that it's possible the restaurant found they could get more work out of Hispanic people than other types of people."

It was obvious the "type" he was talking about. He implied that he thought black men did not deserve these jobs. I had heard this man make subtle racist comments in the past, but what really surprised me was that not one person but myself disagreed with what he said. Because of this and other observations related to rising rates of crime, unemployment, and drug abuse, I thought to myself then—more than twenty years ago—that we as a country were in serious trouble.

I remember walking out of that restaurant with such a weak feeling in my stomach. Here was a group of well-educated, well-intentioned people whose beliefs were inherently racist, and they didn't even realize it. It was a prime example of the invisible hand of racism at work.

Since that time a lot of things, including attitudes, have changed. With the help of integration and affirmative action, people have become more aware of racial issues. Also in that time integration and affirmative action helped create a significant population of middle-class African-Americans.

But a decline in blue collar and retail jobs in inner cities and years of Republican leadership intent on cutting many valuable social programs have also helped create a sizable underclass. The underclass, as it is referred to by some sociologists, developed in the late 1960s and 1970s and is defined by households which live below the poverty level. It comprises 4.5 million African-Americans in the United States.

The plight of the black underclass and the status of the middle-class African-American community are areas of interest to writer and black scholar Dr. William Julius Wilson. Racism and discrimination, which fuel the underclass, are discussed in his latest book, *When Work Disap-*

pears: The World of the New Urban Poor. Wilson interviewed employers at Chicago area companies and discovered that most of them avoided hiring blacks from low-income neighborhoods because they believed that blacks were lazy, dishonest, inarticulate, and uncooperative. One white employer said:

> I think today there is more bias and prejudice against the black man than there was twenty years ago. I think twenty years ago, fifteen years ago, ten years ago, white male employers like myself were willing to give anybody and everybody the opportunity, not because it was the law, but because it was the right thing to do, and today I see more prejudice and racial bias in employers than ever before. . . . [W]hen we hear other employers talk, they'll go after primarily . . . the Mexican, Hispanic, and any Oriental.

Like my experience in the restaurant twenty years ago, the hiring of other ethnic groups besides blacks has become a more recognizable and immediate problem in today's work force. It is a major factor that contributes to stress in the African-American community.

Wilson's depiction of life on the South Side of Chicago could be the story of almost any major city with a significant black population: Newark, Washington, D.C., East St. Louis are a few examples. Whenever I ride through my childhood neighborhoods in West Philadelphia, I am overwhelmed by the number of boarded-up houses and businesses, the vacant lots and trash-strewn streets. I remember when I was not even a teenager walking by myself to the corner grocery store on hot summer afternoons to buy milkshakes and pretzel rods. After school, my girl friends and I would eat kosher pickles and jump rope. Back then the neighborhood may not have been perfect, but it was a safe haven and it was thriving. And what's more, the place felt like a *community.* People of all income levels lived together in harmony. We understood the value of hard work. We had role models to help us. And we had hope. But now, with the decay of the local economy and the onslaught of drug abuse, the sense of togetherness has long departed from these streets. My old neighborhood has become, like so many other cities in this country, a wasteland without growth, hope, and opportunity.

For instance, Wilson points out that in a section of Chicago called

North Lawndale, where there is an African-American population of 60,000, there are only one bank and one supermarket. Yet North Lawndale has forty-eight state lottery agents, fifty check-cashing establishments, and ninety-nine licensed liquor stores and bars.

The result of this social disorganization is obvious. For some, hard work is no longer valued. And responsibility is just a word. Female-headed households dominate the African-American community, and the majority of them are poor. Too often, one adult (usually the mother) bears the responsibility for the social, educational, moral, spiritual, and cultural guidance of her children. To make matters worse, she may likely be responsible for her family's financial demands as well. Within the immediate community, there is a lack of positive role models, including models for intimacy, love, and conflict.

Poverty is stressful. Lack of education is stressful. Job discrimination is stressful. Violence is stressful. Fear, depression, distrust, and isolation only encourage poor health habits. And unfortunately, with daily burdens and stresses, too many do not take the time and energy to eat well, reduce stress, and practice good health habits. Under these conditions, the onslaught of physical disease is inevitable. And so the stress continues.

The Stress of Duality

Middle- and upper-class blacks are not exempt from stress. It is just a different form, more insidious and subtle than that experienced by the underclass. The novelist James Baldwin said that being black in America means you have to be schizophrenic. Other African-Americans have noted this schizophrenic pattern. At the beginning of the century, W.E.B. Du Bois described the African-American psyche: "One ever feels his two-ness—an American, a Negro; two souls, two thoughts, two unreconciled strivings; two warring ideals in one dark body, whose dogged strength alone keeps it from being torn asunder." Du Bois wrote this at the beginning of the century. Almost one hundred years later, this duality has not been resolved.

African-Americans must choose to be one or the other: African-American or American. No other ethnic group in this country is faced with such a choice. If viewed as too Afrocentric or anti-American, Afri-

can-Americans are labeled racist, or at the very least viewed as a threat
to society. Yet other people are allowed to be Irish and American or
Japanese and American or Italian and American. They have willfully
immigrated to this country and, thus, are allowed to have a sense of
pride and honor about their culture. African-Americans have been discouraged from preserving a true cultural identity ever since the first
slave ships arrived in America.

Middle- and upper-class African-Americans exist always in two
worlds, never forgetting the heritage, always mindful of the status, inherited through the centuries. Some African-Americans are careful to
use correct language and pronunciation and not too much black language. Juggling lives between being African-American and American,
not wanting to be noticed while being and feeling excluded. Struggling
daily to be part of humanity; to be seen as children of God.

I have felt my own duality for most of my life. I was the only black
person in my first-grade class, one of only a handful of blacks in my
high school, the only black person in my department at the University
of Pennsylvania, and the only black person in the entire Bastyr University for my first two years. During my studies at the University of Pennsylvania, I was ashamed when I listened to professors explain that blacks
had more criminal tendencies than other ethnic groups because they
believed blacks had smaller brains.

I remember during my studies at John Bastyr how I felt embarrassed
to ask questions because I did not want to appear stupid. After all, as
the only black student in my class, I carried the burden of representing
my entire race. Everything I said and did would be used by my fellow
students and possibly my professors to pass judgment on other black
people. I felt I had to know more and be better than my Caucasian
colleagues. But it hurt me that I thought I was not as smart or as good
as they. I remember the sting I felt inside when a white student asked if
she could touch my hair, or when another classmate said he wanted to
be my friend because of my color. I remember feeling isolated as I
walked the streets of Seattle, which at that time had an 8 percent black
population.

All throughout my levels of education, I felt a peculiar estrangement
from other students and at the same time a need to be one of them, to
be accepted in order to dispel their racial stereotypes of black people.

It is this duality of being black in America that adds to the stress that is felt every day of our lives. Being self-conscious all the time is stressful.

STRESS IN THE WORKPLACE

The stress I experienced at the University of Pennsylvania and John Bastyr is similar to what happens to African-Americans in the workplace. We are afraid to speak up in a group for fear of appearing stupid. We wonder if we are competent or smart enough. Too many patients say things to me like: "Work is so stressful. I'm the only minority in my workplace and they treat me differently. I think it's just the way they were raised. It's very subtle. It makes me lose my confidence. You know there are just subtle things that go with being a minority. I get an award every year but every position I apply for a white female gets the job. Something is just not right." We are forever conscious of our race in a predominantly white workplace environment.

According to researchers George Davis and Glegg Watson, black managers say they feel a special kind of stress due to corporate racism: a subtly worded memo, a missed promotion or work bonus, a supervisor who withholds information, or an unfair evaluation. If racism is no longer working out in the open thanks to civil rights laws, it is still working as an invisible hand, and no place is this hand more menacingly felt than in the workplace.

There is a pervasive feeling that premium positions in corporate America and in the federal government are for whites only. It was not until ten years after the passage of the Civil Rights Act of 1964 that we began to see more African-Americans in managerial positions. This change came about as a result of riots as well as the creation of the Equal Employment Opportunity Commission (EEOC). For the first time, corporations and universities were forced to provide a place for African-Americans.

But all is not well and fair in corporate America. Consider the Texaco lawsuit that attracted attention in November 1996. Top executives at Texaco were recorded on tape using racial epithets to describe African-American employees. "Black jelly beans" was used to refer to the company's attempts to hire more blacks to diversify the racial mix.

"Porch monkey" was used to refer to any highly visible black employee who makes the company appear to have a diversified upper-level management. The use of these and other terms dehumanized blacks once again, and demonstrated that even in the 1990s, well over a century after slavery was abolished, people still viewed African-Americans as objects or animals. In June 1996, the EEOC found that Texaco had discriminated against African-Americans as a class. Yet in November of that same year the chairman of Texaco claimed in the media to be shocked and surprised by the events.

Although affirmative action programs have increased the number of black professionals, the Bureau of Labor Statistics reports that only 4 percent of all managers are black. Texaco, for example, has 19,554 employees, 22.3 percent of whom are black. Yet there are no African-American department heads or vice-presidents. This type of racial glass ceiling, common among large American corporations, creates this scarcity of blacks and adds to the stress of culture shock, isolation, invisibility, and loss of identity. Blacks often act a certain way so that whites will be comfortable even though blacks are never fully accepted by them. But this behavior often creates division among blacks. Patricia J. Williams, one of ten black women who graduated from Harvard Law School in 1975, wrote of her and her colleagues' experiences in all-white firms in a recent *New Yorker* article. My own experiences confirm her comments:

> We have to be more assertive to be invited to the lunch meetings to which our white counterparts are automatically included. The more assertive and successful we are, the more we are exceptional and different from other blacks according to our white colleagues.

Whether in a high-ranking government or corporate managerial position, African-Americans who succeed at work can easily become angry from the stress of juggling work and family responsibilities. One patient I treated had ulcerative colitis, a bowel condition that includes frequent, painful, bloody stools and sometimes requires removal of the entire colon. "Marcia" told me her condition was exacerbated by the stress of being a single parent, the stress of her work demands, and the responsibility of taking care of her healthy mother's livelihood. She had been the family caretaker since childhood. That role fostered grief, anxiety, and resentment.

"I'm always in a position where others demand things from me, even when it's not my responsibility," she confided in me soon after she had been diagnosed with her condition by her allopathic physician.

"Like what?"

"My husband doesn't help me raise my child. My mother demands too much from me. All of my relationships are burdensome, not supportive. I'm not doing what I need for *myself*."

Feeling "unloved, misunderstood, and neglected" are the words used by another patient, "Lisa," to express her anger and resentment toward her family, for whom she bears financial and emotional responsibility.

"I'm angry at Mom for being passive, for not taking control of her life," Lisa told me. "She's dependent on me, but always so negative. I want her to take more control of her life."

When I asked her if she was experiencing any problems at work, she told me she had just received a poor evaluation from her immediate superior. She thought it was unfair.

"I am the only black person with a position of authority in my office. My boss is white—her comments were constructed to trash my reputation and performance."

She had been in her position for eight years and with the company for the past eleven. Fortunately, Lisa was assertive enough to go to the director of her division, who reevaluated her work and changed her evaluation. But she told me she still had self-doubts and felt the enormous pressure to perform better than any of her other colleagues because of her race.

"I know what I'm doing, but I question if it's good enough. Am I projecting the right image?"

In the professional world, Lisa and many other black women often feel a unique type of stress because their status in the company is as a "double minority," or "twofer." White colleagues may view an African-American woman's position in a company as a handout, a way for the company to simultaneously inflate its female and minority percentages. This attitude affects self-confidence. Once again, black women are treated like objects, underpaid, disrespected, and sexually harassed. Taking a firm stand as Lisa did with her director may not diminish the unfairness experienced in other offices in America as immediately. But not taking a stand will surely increase feelings of unworthiness. African-American women will remain in lower-paying positions and continue to lose belief in themselves.

African-Americans are often the last hired and the first fired. In an era of layoffs, "early outs," and downsizing, there is a constant threat of unemployment. Whether real or perceived, racism is the greatest contributor to stress in the workplace. And this stress can lead to sickness. Disease results in a variety of health problems peculiar to the black community, for example, higher rates of hypertension and lower life expectancy. Life expectancy for black men is 64 years versus 70.6 for white men and 72.7 years for black women versus 78.2 for white women.

New studies show that racism inflicts biological stress on black Americans, regardless of their income levels. Other long-term studies have shown that black adults who report high incidences of racism have the most doctor-verified health problems and disabilities. And what of the less serious dis-eases—insomnia, anxiety, headaches, dizziness, and fatigue—for which conventional medicine cannot find a cause? The cause may be stress. The solution is change.

NECESSARY CHANGES

Responsibility has been replaced by a sense that America's debt to us is unpaid. There are many reasons for this, no doubt, reasons which are not due solely to African-Americans. But whatever the reasons, we are suffering. We *are* owed something. But to continue to wait for the collection of this debt is the role we play in our own demise. We owe something to ourselves, our ancestors, and our children—to increase the quality of our lives.

African-Americans must understand and use the history of this country to create a positive self-identity. Stress results from not knowing who you are. This is not new information. The movement in the sixties was specifically directed to being "black and proud." There is much talent and strength in the African-American community. Having survived the atrocities of American history attests to that. African ancestors were forced here, and their children were born under the most devastating circumstances. Many still excel. From Frederick Douglass and Thurgood Marshall, Romare Bearden and Jacob Lawrence, to Michael Jordan, Jackie Joyner Kersey, and Gail Deavers, some are exceptional, but not all: all are ordinary children of God, blessed with talents they chose to develop and use. There are many "exceptions" in the African-American community, but all cannot be exceptions. The people noted above loved and respected themselves enough to do what they loved. They knew who they were as people and as African-Americans.

Some of us have not chosen to do the best we can and some have not been allowed. Talents are gifts from God. But strength and conviction must be used to push through obstacles and make dreams come true. To acquire this dream requires courage and discipline. To rise against odds enhances character and self-esteem. Start here with acknowledgment of your power and your ability to survive and excel, to build an awareness that you are capable of greatness. Escape the boundaries you define and those which others define for you. Learn to love yourself despite the strife, fear, racial discrimination, and stress encountered on a daily basis. We should think of our grandmothers, who did not labor in their domestic jobs so that we could do drugs and alcohol or eat junk food. They did not work fifteen hours a day so that we could abuse ourselves and others. We must hold fast to the knowledge that we too are inheritors of a history that exemplifies strength and greatness. Our ancestors labored and died so that we might have opportunity to do better, so that we can think, "I can do this; I can endure and overcome obstacles until my dream is realized."
END OF SPECIAL NOTE

Think Different Thoughts, Do Different Things: Revolution

We must stop negative thought patterns that bind us to the idea that we are not good enough, that we are not smart enough. The more we think this way, the more susceptible we are to dis-ease. Thoughts are powerful, and negative thoughts in particular are addictive, habitual, and stressful. From an early age we hear negatives: "Stop." "Don't." "No." We tell our children, "Don't drop the vase," rather than "Hold on to the vase." The messages are very different. One is comforting and instructive; the other is demanding and stressful. We could choose affirmative, comforting messages in our lives. We also think negatively about who we are and what we can and cannot do. Condescending phrases like "I am so stupid" or "I can't do that" can easily become self-fulfilling beliefs.

It is heartening, however, to see a recent major shift in consciousness in this country. People seem to be taking more responsibility for themselves. They seem to be caring more for others, too. One example is in the increased interest and support for complementary medicine, which emphasizes patient responsibility and involvement in their health care. One way African-American men responded to this shift was the Million Man March in October 1995. Americans must continue to be part of this movement toward claiming more responsibility for ourselves, our behaviors, our lives, and our health. In the midst of fighting and hatred, some are learning forgiveness and love. We must, for example, learn to love the intentions of our parents and forgive their often flawed methods. Many of us are letting go of old hurts and anger and learning to live more in the moment. This attitude filters into families and communities and has the potential to effect a significant change.

For African-Americans, living in the moment means we need not blame present problems on white people who lived hundreds of years ago. African-Americans are not absolved of the responsibility to make something of this life because of the legacy of slavery. Likewise Caucasian Americans need also to live in the present and not continue to apply old stereotypes and discriminatory behavior toward people of color. Maybe our children's children will see an end to bigotry, racism, and discrimination, but we will not. Racism will exist, slavery will always be a painful memory. But we cannot help the cause by contributing to our own demise. We must change. It is time for a *real* revolution.

In my late teens and early twenties I talked and read a lot about revolution: revolting against the way things were, against the American system, against white people. I grew up at a time when the Black Panthers, Angela Davis, and the Honorable Elijah Muhammad talked of African-Americans separating from white America, for the most part by force. I never considered then that I would be part of a revolution. Though what they said about the racial dynamics of this country was true, I was not willing to hurt or destroy another human being because of the color of his skin or his opposing beliefs. Violence was never an option.

Revolution requires a radical departure from business as usual. Revolution can be personal: changing what goes on inside ourselves, a revolt against the constant hatred for whom we have been taught to believe we are, revolution against the hatred of white people just because they are white or against the hatred of black people because they are black. Think what a powerful force this could be for the advancement of humankind.

The revolution must begin within each of us, and it must begin now. We need to recognize, for example, that life is precious, and we ought to exercise control over it. We must create a sense of self, inclusion, wellness, and freedom. We must, each of us that knows the truth, no matter what color, be responsible for the re-membering of the human race. We can have wellness if we have wholeness. There is much work to be done and we need to be well to do it.

You are what you know. It does not matter what you believe you are. Empty your mind of negative beliefs and let the truth replace them. The truth is that we are all children of God. You are a daughter or son of God. God will give you anything. But you have to let God know what you want, what is important to you, by your actions. What you want is already yours; no one can take it away from you. There is so much support for each of us if we choose to use it and seek it out. God does not just drop you on earth and say, "Now let's see what you can do alone."

It doesn't matter which God you believe in. You can accept these simple facts. God is not somewhere in heaven. God is in everything, everyone, everywhere. We are made in God's image. As children of this Spirit, we are entitled to abundant joy. We are entitled to good mental, emotional, and physical health. We must reconcile ourselves to this fact.

We must dispel the illusion of separate races. We are all one people. We are not bodies; we are our spirits. The body is a way to experience life on earth. We need our bodies to learn and grow, and we need an ego to let us distinguish between ourselves and others. By the same token, being different is not the same as being separate from one another and from God. In spirit, no one is better than another. We may differ in the way we behave, but we ought not to judge others' behavior. We don't have to like it, or participate in it, but to judge another is a sin.

Stress results from believing we are wrong or have made mistakes. There are no mistakes. Whatever we have done, we did because we put our trust in something other than the truth or we chose to ignore what we knew to be correct. All experience can be summed up in three basic lessons:

- ❧ Love God—in everything, everyone, everywhere—with all your heart, mind, body, and soul.
- ❧ Love your neighbor as yourself (this presumes we know how to love ourselves first).
- ❧ Forgive yourself and others for judging behavior as wrong.

God will provide experiences and circumstances so we can learn lessons. Whether it is through an act of racism or an act of loving, we are here to learn to love one another. The fact that most people do not love themselves is, in itself, stressful. Self-deprecating behavior takes many forms, such as an abusive relationship or a job we hate, and is invariably related to low self-esteem. We say we want a positive whole-some relationship or a career in which we can use our skills and talents, but we do not demonstrate the seriousness of these desires. We do not create ways to fulfill them. We say we want to eat well and lose weight, yet we continue to buy foods that have no nutritional value and are high in fat and sugar. We give ourselves mixed messages. Our actions and behavior don't match. We say we want X but we do Y. Say "Yes" when you mean yes and "No" when you mean no. Stand up for what you believe is best for you, not what you think someone else would like you to do. Be assertive. Read books and take self-realization courses or seminars to teach you to be firm in a loving way. Feel empowered to make choices. Freedom is a choice. If you are reading this book, you are on the way to freedom, to raising your consciousness about who you are. Living fully is a choice. Good health is a choice. Loving ourselves and others is a choice.

If you have not already done so, you must forgive yourself for judging yourself and comparing yourself to others. You must never accept the belief that you are not as good as other people. One way to change these negative judgments is to practice prayer, affirmations, and forgiveness. We affirm our prayers.

Forgiveness is a major step toward stress reduction and wellness. It must come from the heart and not be only an intellectual exercise.

Forgiveness allows us to have freedom from anger, sadness, and guilt. When we have freedom from negative emotions, we are able to love and be joyful.

Spend time every day creating affirmations. They should indicate action and be written in the first person. Here are examples: *"I am forgiving myself for judging myself as wrong."* Or, *"I am forgiving myself for judging myself as inadequate."*

Create meaningful affirmations that speak to your issues. Then practice saying them every day. Begin by taking slow, deep breaths for two minutes in order to relax. If you need to, put fifty toothpicks on the floor. As you say each affirmation, move a toothpick to the side until you've created another pile with all fifty toothpicks. Also, you might carry a card with several affirmations to read during the day.

Each of us has roles to play in God's plan. The spirit's job is to assist us in discovering and performing them. Through discipline and repeated contact with spirit, we find our roles in life. And in order to achieve this discipline and contact, we should sit down every day to reflect on our breathing and communicate with the God within us. You may choose to light a candle and watch the flame while you focus on your breathing. Do not try to clear your mind. Just focus on your breath and your thoughts will drift. At the beginning, you may be able to do this for only ten minutes, but in time you will have the discipline to sit for a half hour or more every day. Continue the exercise even if you don't perceive a difference in yourself. Others will see the difference, and you will notice changes in the way they react to you.

As with learning anything new, we need to break old habits and create new ones. We have to step through fear and replace it with loving. It is also critical to have faith that God does not give us a role without the means to fulfill it. God does not give us more than we can handle. We are not meant to be unhappy. Confronting our fears is the only way to break them. We must be revolutionary in our thinking, speaking, vision, and behavior. We must empower ourselves. We must take care of ourselves by creating healthier lifestyles for our minds, bodies, and souls.

The following are some guidelines that are elements of a personal growth seminar called "Insight," in which I participated in the early eighties, and which I now share with my patients.

- ❧ Take care of yourself so you can take care of others.
- ❧ Do not hurt yourself or others.
- ❧ Use everything to your advancement.

Only when we sincerely take care of ourselves and become content with who we are can we create peace and congeniality with others. In doing so we maintain our health and integrity and we put ourselves in a better position to take care of others without expecting anything in return. In my experience, independence and willingness to stand up for ourselves encourage others to do the same. We need a variety of changes in our behavior to reduce stress and begin a private revolution. To change what you get, you must change who you are. Small things done consistently over time create major changes. Do the following things consistently.

- ❧ Be gentle with yourself.
- ❧ Do something for yourself each day that gives you strength and vitality.
- ❧ Exercise regularly.
- ❧ Enjoy the moment.
- ❧ Focus on the blessings in your life. Take time at the end of the day to record in a journal what you are grateful for and the good things that have happened during the day. Also record the good things you did during the day. Remembering our good things increases our self-esteem.
- ❧ Take time to be with nature and people who love and support you.
- ❧ Take relaxation breaks. Learn a variety of relaxation techniques (visualization, meditation) and practice at least one regularly.
- ❧ Do one thing at a time, keeping your mind focused on the present. Do whatever you are doing more slowly, more intentionally, and with more awareness.
- ❧ Simplify your life. Eliminate experiences and people who do not support your growth.
- ❧ Organize your life to include fun and spontaneous activities. Create a realistic schedule. Eliminate unnecessary commitments (say "No" when you mean no).

- ❧ Do unpleasant tasks immediately rather than worry about them all day.
- ❧ Do not expect yourself and others to be different from what you (they) really are.
- ❧ Forgive yourself for judging yourself and others as wrong.
- ❧ Laugh more often.
- ❧ Practice communication skills such as using "I" statements. Empowerment can come through changing "I need" to "I want" and "I have to" to "I choose to." For example, you don't have to go to work; you choose to go to work so that you can afford to live the way you have chosen. If you don't, the consequences will lower your self-esteem and sense of security.
- ❧ Choose neither to waste the present with guilt over the past nor to worry about the future, because in this moment neither exists. Be here now.
- ❧ Take slow deep breaths often, especially in your car and when waiting for something or someone. Notice people and say out loud, if need be, "That is God."
- ❧ Finish something, anything.

Practicing self-love and self-respect, and responding to life with integrity and responsibility, will reduce the amounts of stress. If we look within ourselves for empowerment and purpose, we can know the meaning of wellness. If each of us has a positive personal revolution that stills our internal voices and forces of oppression, we can permeate this country and our world with a dignity and hope that we have never experienced in our lives. Let us have an American Revolution.

6

HYPERTENSION

In the late 1980s, Dr. Clarence E. Grim, professor of medicine and director of the Charles R. Drew Hypertension Renal Clinic at UCLA, released a theory that the higher rate of hypertension among African-Americans was due to the genetic characteristics of African slaves who survived the "middle" passage to America. Dr. Grim estimated that 45 to 50 percent of all slaves died from vomiting, diarrhea and general fluid (mineral) loss as a result of this experience. Those who survived were slaves whose kidneys retained excessive amounts of salt and water.

Other researchers say this theory does not consider an important factor: stress—especially the stress of living in the inner city. The stress of poor socioeconomic living conditions, high rates of unemployment and underemployment, crime, poverty, and racial discrimination are also variables that cannot be overlooked when addressing the question of our higher rates of hypertension. We know that chronic stress makes the nervous system release norepinephrine, a hormone that causes the kidneys to slow down the elimination of salt.

Researchers at Johns Hopkins have had similar ideas. If the laws of genetics bear any truth, then African-Americans with darker skin should have inherited more of their genes from dark-skinned West African ancestors. But what these researchers at Hopkins found was that blacks with darker skin and higher blood pressure also ranked low in their socioeconomic status, or did not finish high school; high blood pressure is not only a matter of skin color.

Dr. Grim and other researchers could be correct. It is possible that African-Americans have a predisposition to hypertension because of the conditions suffered by slaves. But we also know that stress can temporarily raise anyone's blood pressure. I have a personal story to tell you that illustrates this connection.

When I first opened my practice in Washington, D.C., in 1988, people often did not keep their appointments or even call to cancel. Because my first appointment with a new patient is an hour and a half, the missed appointments were leading to a considerable waste of time and money. I asked my friend and mentor how to resolve this problem. He told me to require a deposit for each new patient. And that was the beginning of the deposit policy in my office.

When a new patient calls, the receptionist explains our policy. If a deposit is not received within two weeks of the scheduled visit, the name is erased from my book and that slot is filled by someone on my waiting list. The deposit is, of course, credited to the initial visit fee. My staff calls every patient to confirm two days before and then one day before the visit. The staff then puts a red check mark beside the patient's name to let me know he or she is coming.

One day, in the fall of 1996, I asked my receptionist to call the next new patient on my schedule because she had not yet arrived. Cheryl came into my office to tell me the new patient was on the phone and was confused about the appointment, even though she had returned my receptionist's call the day before to confirm the appointment. After we exchanged introductions, the woman explained that she had made the appointment for her son. She told me she got confused when Cheryl called the day before because she thought it was for another doctor with the same last name. And even though she called us back, she did not realize the difference in phone numbers or addresses at the time of confirmation. She said when she called the other doctor's office that day, the receptionist there said they did not have a scheduled appointment. She did not think to call my office.

Part of it had to do with me and part of it was in the way she was explaining herself, but I was simply confused by her story. When I asked her to repeat herself, the woman changed her story. She said the other doctor's name was not the same as mine. Even though we were forty-five minutes into her appointment time, I offered to allow her to come in immediately to begin the interview process, but she refused. She wanted to make another appointment, but she did not want to pay another deposit fee. I told her, given the circumstances, I would not be willing to change the rules for her. If she wanted to make another appointment, she would have to pay another deposit fee.

This woman suddenly became hostile over the phone. She began yelling and saying, "Who do you think you are?" I told her I was sorry for the confusion but that I was not willing to talk to her anymore if she was going to be offensive. Ten minutes later her husband called back. He began the conversation by asking bluntly, "What have you done to upset my wife? She said you were rude and unpleasant to her." I told him what had happened and that his wife was already upset when we called her. I assured him I was neither rude nor unpleasant. He threatened me by telling me he knew a lot of people in Washington and he could see to it that they would never come to my office. He also threatened to write the Better Business Bureau. I told him I was sorry for the confusion and that he was entitled to do whatever he thought he should do.

Then it happened.

He said, "You're black, aren't you? You're a black doctor?"

I asked him what difference it made whether I was white or black. Without answering me, he asked again and then said, "I know you black people, you black doctors. You come from *nothing* and think you are something. But you are *nothing* and you come from *nothing*." Then he began to curse at me. I calmly told him I was not willing to engage in any further conversation with him and that I was hanging up the phone. And that's what I did.

Though I do not suffer from hypertension, I know my blood pressure was elevated. I could feel my face flushing with blood, and my heart racing, as if I was about to explode. I realized I was also shaking. I felt assaulted by the hatred in his voice and frightened by the evil of racism. I calmed down, eventually, by thinking of my ancestors and knowing I did come from *something*.

I believe that, because the stress of being black in America is so permanent and consistent, the susceptibility to hypertension is constantly magnified. Over time the ability to normalize the pressure is lost. Some researchers have shown that the experience of racial discrimination subjects people to demeaning, stressful and perhaps violent situations that may contribute to poor health. Persons who have experienced greater incidences of racism and are less acculturated to European culture are more likely to smoke and have higher blood pressure than those who are more acculturated. Those persons who are discriminated against hold negative self-evaluations and participate in negative health habits such as excessive drinking, smoking, drug abuse, and eating. In addition, our poor dietary habits add stress to our physical bodies, thereby increasing our susceptibility to hypertension.

Whether it is suppressed anger, low self-esteem, or socioeconomic status that does in fact contribute to hypertension, we should acknowledge that these conditions at the very least are stressful and constant. And one thing is clear: hypertension is due to many factors, not just one. Some of these factors involve racism, abuse, socioeconomics, genetics, weight, and diet, and each requires a treatment that is equally diverse.

WHAT IS HYPERTENSION?

Hypertension occurs when the smaller blood vessels (arterioles) that branch off from the arteries become constricted and impede blood flow. As a result, blood pressure rises and forces the heart to work harder. A person has hypertension when his blood pressure checks in consistently at 140/90 mm Hg. The top figure is called the systolic pressure and indicates the pressure the heart exerts at the time it is pumping, or at work. The bottom figure is called the diastolic pressure and indicates the pressure in the heart when it is at rest. Acute severe hypertension occurs when the diastolic pressure is greater than 150 mm Hg. Usually the person will also experience symptoms of headache or blurred vision. If this is your experience, it is an emergency situation and you should receive immediate medical attention.

There are two categories of hypertension: primary—or essential—and secondary. More than 90 percent of all cases of hypertension are primary or their cause is unknown. Certain factors aggravate the condition. African-Americans, for instance, have higher incidences of hypertension. It is also more common among men, anyone over thirty-five, obese people, and smokers. Also, if you suffer from diabetes mellitus, hypercholesterolemia, cardiac enlargement, congestive heart failure, or myocardial infarction, you are at greater risk. Other factors include high blood sodium to potassium ratio, high sugar/low fiber diets, high unsaturated fatty acids/low saturated fatty acids diets, frequent alcohol consumption, and diets low in calcium, magnesium, and vitamin C.

Secondary hypertension describes a condition of high blood pressure that is the result of some other medical condition, like kidney failure, renal artery stenosis (constriction of the arteries that lead to the kidneys), hyperthyroidism (overactive thyroid gland), and adrenal gland disease. Other causes of secondary hypertension are drugs, such as anabolic steroids, oral contraceptives, cocaine or crack, and amphetamines. And finally, alcohol withdrawal, as well as acute pain and acute stress, can also contribute to hypertension.

Hypertension is another disease naturopaths believe is associated with the Western diet. More commonly found in developed countries, people in New Guinea, Brazil, Africa, and Panama, for example, have almost no experience of essential hypertension. One in four Americans has hypertension. But somewhere between 30 to 40 percent of black Americans suffer from this condition. According to the American Heart Association, blacks are twice as likely to have hypertension as whites, five to seven times more likely to have chronic hypertension, and three to five times more likely to suffer from cardiovascular mortality. (Black males under the age of forty-five are ten times more likely to die from hypertension—or suffer the debilitating strokes that often come with it—than white males of the same age. African-Americans also have an increased risk of cardiac enlargement, end-stage renal disease (which leads to hypertension), and stroke. Thus, based on these figures, black males overall are ten times more likely to die of high blood pressure (or suffer from strokes associated with hypertension) than white males of the same age.

The case you are about to read is of a woman I will call Helen. She came to me already on medication for hypertension and for treatment of a benign ovarian cyst. When she came to visit, she was comfortable with the drug and wanted me to help treat her cyst, which was over six centimeters in diameter and periodically caused her pain.

During her first interview I quickly learned that she had lost her husband six months before. She began crying as she talked about how angry she was with herself for not having spoken to him the day he passed away. She continued to weep when she told me she had known he was ill but had not done anything to help him. Several years before, he had had a heart attack, followed by congestive heart failure. Not surprisingly, he was overweight and had poor eating habits. She worked at night, but they briefly talked in the morning before he left for the office. But on the morning he died she did not wake up to see him off. When she called him at noon, he had been taken to the hospital. He never regained consciousness.

Helen told me she was a controlling person and thought at first she would do whatever was necessary to make arrangements for the funeral and put her finances in order. After that, she would grieve, stay home awhile, and then move on with her life. But she realized she felt guilty and angry with herself. She couldn't shake those feelings. Despite attending support groups and praying every day, she still felt helpless. "I had no control over this," she said.

Helen talked a lot about her marriage and her work, and described herself in both contexts as being driven, impatient, and argumentative. Because of her drive, her self-anger, her controlling and argumentative nature, and her impatience, I prescribed the remedy nux vomica in a 200 c potency to treat her temperament and stimulate her body to heal itself.

After two months her mood and temperament had become more pleasant and balanced. She was no longer impatient or quarrelsome. Her cyst had reduced in size and her sleep habits had improved. She changed her diet, which consisted of lots of chocolate, tuna fish, white bread, coffee and coffee creamer, and limited fruits and vegetables, to the diet recommended in Chapter 4, "Nutrition and Your Blood Type"—high in fiber and complex carbohydrates, with lots of fish for her type O blood. Helen took a multivitamin and the herbs gelsemium, phytolacca, Bryonia, and aconitum for the cyst. After five months she was much better in every respect, except she was still smoking. I gave her a combination of lobelia, valerian, scutellaria, and cayenne and increased her exercise regimen. She returned in eight months and announced she had stopped smoking and had decided to go back to school. I wished her well.

CASE I

I didn't realize then that I wouldn't see her again for another one and a half years. It was only then that I learned of her feelings during her childhood and how that period of her life created the susceptibility to hypertension.

After a warm exchange of greetings, Helen said to me, "I have not been following the diet and I have been feeling badly about myself and school." When I asked her what that meant, she gave me the big picture.

The classes she was taking for a master's in teaching were beyond full capacity, which meant that assistance and supplies were limited. She was growing frustrated about the situation and complained to the appropriate administrators on several occasions. They told her nothing could be done about the situation. During one meeting, when the administrators did not appear to be concerned about her requests, she suddenly became angry and "blew up." She went to the nurse's office after the incident and found that her blood pressure was up to 180/110 mm Hg. And since that day her blood pressure had not gone down very much.

With all of the time she spent trying to resolve these administrative issues, Helen quickly fell behind in her classwork. She began feeling badly about herself and wondered if she really was capable of finishing school. Her self-confidence was very low. "I don't think I'm good enough to complete the program," she told me.

Whenever a patient makes a statement like that, I need to know where that feeling is coming from and what it means exactly. So I said, "Tell me about that feeling. . . . Where does it come from?"

She immediately responded, "My childhood. There was no encouragement for me as a child. I felt bad 'cause I was dark and ugly."

Helen had a half brother, and she remembered when they were introduced to someone in school the person said, "You aren't his sister. Why do you have nappy hair and he has good hair?" She was ashamed and embarrassed by the way she looked. She did not see any beauty in dark people. She cried all the time and was teased often about her looks. In essence, she hated herself.

"I never had any plans about where I wanted to be when I grew up," she said. "I felt bad that I didn't have any plans." But her household provided little support for her future goals. Her mother used to say to her, "You can't pour piss out of a boot. You can't do a thing." Without any encouragement or guidance from her family, she dropped out of school at age fifteen to marry an abusive nineteen-year-old man.

He abused her mentally and physically, but she remained with him for twelve long years, mainly because of the children, she said. She even stayed with him knowing that he was the father of a child with another woman.

Because she did not finish high school, Helen worried that people with college degrees would see a deficiency in her or think she was stupid. She didn't think they would want to be with her and so she avoided people and remained quiet when she was in a group. She seldom thought she had anything to contribute to any group.

Helen's profile makes perfectly clear the stress of being black in America. The low self-esteem, the suppressed anger, and the insecurity and self-hatred because of her color led to a susceptibility to dis-ease. In this case, those feelings, combined with poor dietary habits and lack of exercise, created the disease of hypertension. Having this understanding of her condition, I prescribed the remedy Lac caninum in a 200 c potency.

Her diet, while much improved from her first visit over a year before, still had too many white sugar and white flour products, as well as too many foods high in salt and fat. I put her back on the detoxification diet for a ten-day period, followed by the strict diet for her O blood type. Because her cholesterol was dangerously high, I also began an herbal and vitamin supplementation. Specifically, I asked her to take a multiple vitamin, garlic, essential fatty acids, lecithin, and rauwolfia. I also told her she had to begin an exercise regimen intended for her blood type. She needed essentially to race-walk, jog, cycle, or jump rope at least four times a week for thirty-five to forty-five minutes, at a moderate pace!

She returned in six weeks and said, "I'm comfortable with school now. I don't feel as though I can't do it. I may have to take more courses before I can get where I want to be, but it doesn't matter. I feel good about myself."

Helen had not been exercising as regularly as I'd suggested, but she was at least working out twice a week. Her blood pressure had lowered to 160/100. As she continued to exercise more frequently and monitor her diet, she watched her pressure continue to drop. But she lacked the discipline necessary to maintain a regular exercise regimen and this had wild effects on her pressure. While she was out of range of acute hypertension, her pressure is still borderline at 140/90.

CASE II

Unfortunately, many of my patients come to me with stories of shame and inferiority. There is too much pain on the planet. Physical abuse is a common tale told behind my closed doors. Usually the story involves a woman who grows up with an abusive father and eventually marries an abusive husband. But the following is a story of a man named William, who also suffered physical abuse.

William was sixty-two when he came to my office. For the past five years he had been suffering from sexual impotence that resulted from taking hypertension medication. Though he had stopped taking the medication over three and a half years ago, he still suffered poor sexual performance.

I asked him to tell me about the stresses in his life, the challenges and issues he had to overcome. He told me the following story. His wife had died one and a half years ago. She had a heart attack in their home and was dead in less than fifteen minutes. He had been married to her for nearly thirty years, and after her death he couldn't even talk about it. He could not go to places where he and his wife used to visit. He could not see friends they knew together. He withdrew gradually from everyone except his closest friends. He stopped working because he could not concentrate. But four months ago he had begun working again as a mechanic because he felt as if he had finally come to terms with his wife's death.

Their marriage had been difficult. For starters, William's wife was very old-fashioned. She believed the husband should be the breadwinner of the house, so she stayed at home. For the last seven months of her life, she would not have anything to do with him. She complained and criticized him about his sexual performance. He had asked her repeatedly to go to the doctor with him to help understand why he was having sexual difficulties, but she refused to go. He felt stressed out all the time because of this situation. Usually when they argued she would hit him, but he never hit back. He would simply stand there and block her blows. To quiet her down, he would have to apologize, even if he was not at fault. Then she would hold a grudge against him for days, sometimes weeks.

William would get angry at his wife, but he would never show it. This character trait also played out at work—he would sometimes get angry at a colleague or his boss, but he would never show this anger. Because he was concerned with doing what was acceptable to others, he often hid his emotions and acted in ways he thought he should.

This demeanor, I learned, was born out of his childhood. His mother would kick him and beat him and tell him he was worthless. "She almost killed me once," he said. "I was so afraid of her. I would do everything I could to stay out of her way. She wouldn't feed me if I did something she didn't like. I might get a peanut butter sandwich for the whole day, and sometimes not that much." Another form of punishment involved putting him in the closet, which was hot and sometimes full of mosquitoes. "We had no fans then. We were poor," he said almost apologetically.

William was also afraid of his father. "When he came home, he took up where she left off. He would draw blood." Despite all of the horrible things he revealed to me, he did not hold any of this against his parents. He did not brood over these events. When he entered the service, he sent most of his money home to his mother. "I did a lot for her. I have no malice." Yet his blood pressure at the time he met me was 150/90.

William's suppression of anger, fear, and insults created a disposition to disease. Rather than expressing anger, he expressed apologies, as if he were ashamed or guilty for feeling this emotion. I could sense that he was a sensitive and gentle man, and this observation, combined with his circumstances, led me to prescribe staphysagria in a 200 c potency.

After ten weeks William returned to my office to say his sleeping habits were much better (an important indicator that the body is trying to heal itself). He had only been sleeping about three and a half hours per night before he came to see me, but now he was sleeping five hours a night. Most importantly, the quality of his sleep had improved. He also had begun walking/jogging forty to fifty minutes a day, as I had requested. His diet was much better and he was more conscious of reading labels and eating foods without additives. He also said he was speaking out more at work. And furthermore, his blood pressure was 140/86. After knowing that his diet, exercise, and remedy were having a positive effect on his condition, I prescribed garlic, because of its ability to lower blood pressure, and herbal preparations.

Three more months passed and when William returned to my office again he said he felt great. He was able to have erections and desires every morning, but his girlfriend was away so he did not have ample opportunity to test his potency. His sleeping habits had improved and his blood pressure had lowered to a respectable 130/86. Over the four years I have known him, I have had to repeat his homeopathic remedy periodically. Throughout that time he has remained on a good multiple vitamin and an herbal combination. I also have had to put him back on the detox diet occasionally and remind him to continue exercising (he is blood type O), but today these lifestyle changes have become his way of life. His blood pressure remains at a steady 130/82.

CASE III

Diane came to my office complaining of low energy, high cholesterol (230) and borderline high blood pressure (140/90). She was in her late twenties and slightly overweight. She also had a story of abuse rejection, poor self-confidence and stress, but not because she is African-American. She and her father had "no relationship." Her father was alcoholic and was never around; he finally left the family when Diane was six. After he left he remarried and had promised to come over to visit or take Diane for the weekend, but he seldom kept his promises. "At some point I was not allowed to call his house because of his new wife. I felt rejected and lousy; I felt really bad about myself, like I wasn't doing things good enough for him to come around or for me to go to his house. When I did see him he would tell me 'Shut up' a lot or he'd make fun of me. He could be vicious with words. Later in life I wrote him to tell him how I felt. He wrote back and essentially told me to get over it. We did not communicate after that. He died and I didn't know he was ill because we hadn't talked in ten years. I was going to call him and then he died," she says, tearing. She felt guilty, saying, "I should have done more; I should have been a better daughter. I feel like I did something wrong."

In relationships Diane always had a fear that the person would leave her because there was something wrong with her. She had conflict about getting close to men for fear they would leave. And when she got close she drove men away from her by being too dependent on them and frightened that they would leave her. "I feel embarrassed and ashamed,

I know it's my fault. I always think people will think I am horrible. I lose my identity in relationships." She was currently in a relationship in which she constantly felt he would leave her. "I get frightened and cry a lot. I have fear that I will never be good enough and be in a good relationship. I always try to avoid conflict and do things for others' approval. Decisions are hard for me because I am always trying to please others."

Diane's history of verbal abuse and parental neglect along with the feeling that she had done something wrong was a source of stress for her at an early age. As she grew into being a young adult she continued the pressure on herself to do the right thing and to please others before herself. She was dependent and in constant need of affection and reassurance. She blamed herself for the pressure she put on men especially but she could not break the cycle. She cried often. The pressure and conflict manifested inside of her created the susceptibility to the cardiovascular conditions of hypertension and high cholesterol.

Her mood, dependency, need for approval, inability to make decisions, frequent crying, other food and temperature preferences suggested that she needed the remedy pulsatilla, which I believed would decrease her moodiness, dependence upon others, and need for approval. I believed this remedy would provide the energy she needed to support and depend upon herself, decrease her tendency to cry, and reduce her high blood pressure. A patient whose mood and emotional state are balanced is more capable of making necessary dietary changes, and Diane was no different.

Diane's diet diary reflected another possible reason why she had high cholesterol: ice cream, cheeses, lots of butter, and pizza. She also ate vegetables and a particular fruit but her diet generally was high in fat and low in complex carbohydrates and fiber. Six weeks after her initial visit, Diane reported, "Overall I feel good; my mood and temperament are really good. I am a little tired but not like before. My sleep is great and I am not sluggish in the morning as I used to be." When I questioned her specifically about the detox diet she said, "Physically I am feeling really healthy too. I had lots more bowel movements and I felt cleaned out."

After three months Diane returned and told me that, even though her work was very stressful because of reduced staff, she was feeling very "positive and strong. I am handling stress a lot better. I fired someone last week I had been wanting to fire but was too uncomfortable to do it. Even with the stress my mood is good. I am speaking my opinion more without being afraid. I have been telling the truth no matter what the person wants to hear. I have been much better at handling others' opinions too." Her relationship was good though she still had some fears that it would not work and she would not marry, but not because he would leave her but rather because it would be by mutual agreement. I had given her a diet for her blood type and she was doing quite well eating in the ways I prescribed.

At the end of six months she and her boyfriend had separated and, while she was saddened by the breakup, she said to me, "It's painful to think about the relationship. I wanted someone to love and care for me. But I have to love and care for myself. And I am doing that now. I just did not and will not suppress myself anymore for anyone." Her blood pressure was normal and her cholesterol was down to 190mg/dl.

I only see Diane every four months now, and during our last visit I learned she decided to quit her job and change careers. While she is dating, she is not looking to be in a relationship so that someone can take care of her. "I am feeling very independent. I am not clingy. I am different. My need for approval is gone. I do not want to give up my life to be with anyone. I am clear that all the stuff around my father is healing."

Herbal Treatments
and Nutritional Supplements

HERBAL PREPARATIONS

There are several ways to use herbs. The preparations most common and readily available are teas, tinctures, infusions, decoctions, tablets, and capsules. I usually prescribe two herbs at a time and sometimes alternate with an additional two.

> ☙ A **decoction** is prepared by adding the herbal formula (usu-
> ally ⅛ ounce of bark or root of the herb) to boiling water
> (usually 4 ounces) and allowing the mixture to simmer for
> three to ten minutes. Then the solution should be allowed
> to steep for ten minutes. During this time, more water is

added to compensate for whatever water has evaporated. The decoction should then be strained and the liquid given to the patient.

✤ **Infusions** may be either hot or cold. Usually the proportions are 1 part herb to 16 to 20 parts water. Though prepared like an herbal tea, infusions are allowed to steep for twenty to thirty minutes to create a more potent solution.

✤ A **tea** is made by steeping 1 tablespoon of fresh dried herbs in 1 cup boiling water for five minutes, then straining the solution.

✤ **Tinctures** are made by soaking the herb in an alcohol solution for at least two weeks. The solution is periodically shaken. The liquid that remains after straining the solution is the tincture. A tincture can also be used to make a tea by adding a prescribed amount of drops to boiling water.

✤ A tincture with all of the alcohol distilled from it becomes an extract, which is a potent concentrate of the herb. **Capsules** and **tablets** can be made from the powder produced by removing all of the moisture from the extract and grinding the concentrate.

The major antihypertensive botanical medicines are *Allium sativaum* (garlic), *Viscum album* (European mistletoe), *Valerian officinalis* (valerian), *Crataegus oxyacantha* (hawthorn berry), *Veratrum viride* (green hellebore), and *Rauwolfia serpentina* (rauwolfia).

Garlic has been used for many conditions for thousands of years. Combined with proper diet and exercise, garlic has some hypotensive qualities—in other words, it helps to reduce both systolic and diastolic pressures. Perhaps more importantly, it reduces fat buildup (cholesterol and triglycerides) in the blood, which further helps reduce blood pressure. I recommend at least one fresh clove (not a bulb!) three times a day, or one 1000 mcg capsule three times a day.

Mistletoe is used in combination with valerian and green hellebore. Viscum has many pharmacological effects. It has demonstrated vasodilating (expanding the smooth muscles of the arteries), hypotensive, and sedative properties, as well as cardiac depressant and antispasmodic properties. But it should be administered carefully. Part of its hypotensive action is to inhibit the excitability of the vasomotor center (the area responsible for regulating the diameter of the blood vessels) in the medulla oblongata of the brain (the lower portion of the brain connected to the spinal column). Please note: **Mistletoe is toxic in large amounts.**

Valerian acts as a sedative in an excited person and a stimulant in a depressed person, thus normalizing the central nervous system. It also helps to lower blood pressure, stimulate the flow of bile (a substance secreted by the liver for the purpose of digesting fats) and relax intestinal muscles. It decreases blood pressure by expanding the arteries of the heart and regulating the heartbeat. I have used it primarily as a hypotensive and sedative for insomnia, as well as a calming agent for the effects of withdrawal from drugs, including alcohol and tobacco.

Green hellebore is also toxic in large doses. But when a person is experiencing headaches and dizziness from hypertension, it can in small doses act as a circulatory depressant, relaxing the heart and slowing the pulse. Veratrum is not to be used for people who are weak, mentally depressed, and/or hypotensive. I mix a tincture of green hellebore with tinctures of mistletoe and valerian in equal parts, and prescribe 20 drops, three times a day.

Because it increases muscle tone, *Crataegus oxyacantha* is an important cardiac tonic and therefore a hypotensive. It contains many constituents that perform a variety of biological activities. It acts to improve the blood flow by expanding the arteries around the heart. Crataegus also improves functional heart activity by improving the heart's metabolism. This herb increases the heart's tolerance to low levels of oxygen and improves athletic performance. It can be combined effectively with mistletoe and the herb rauwolfia. I suggest that patients take 20 drops of crataegus in the morning and before bed.

An Indian physician named Vakil first introduced the herb rauwolfia into practice in 1940. According to Dr. Vakil, the herb was written about in Hindu texts dating back to 1000 B.C. and A.D. 200. In popular medicine it is used as an antidote for snake and insect bites, headaches, anxiety, and abdominal pain. It also has a sedative effect on the nerves. It has been written that Gandhi would drink rauwolfia tea at night if overstimulated by a lecture or argument with someone.

Rauwolfia is a powerful plant, not sold commercially without a doctor's prescription. The most powerful of its many constituents is a substance called reserpine. Its hypotensive effect involves a reduction in heart rate, a contraction of the pupils, and a stimulation of the intestinal peristalsis (waves of muscle contraction and relaxation that allow easier movement of the intestines). Acting primarily on the central nervous system, rauwolfia tends to balance one's emotional state. When taken in small doses, such as the 3–5 drops per day that I prescribe to some patients, the substance has no harmful side effects. But with larger doses come diarrhea and nasal congestion. It is contraindicated in depressed patients.

Nutrients such as sodium, potassium, calcium, magnesium, essential fatty acids, and fiber are all equally as important to this multifaceted approach to treating hypertension. Excessive consumption of sodium chloride, with decreased consumption of dietary potassium, creates an increase in fluid volumes outside of the cells and damages the mechanisms that regulate blood pressure. If an individual is susceptible, this will create hypertension. A high-potassium/low-sodium diet reduces the rise in blood pressure, especially during mental stress and reduces the buildup of fluid volume in cells. This diet benefits several systems in the body that affect blood pressure: the renin-angiotensin system, the aldosterone system, and the sympathetic nervous system (see Glossary for details on these systems).

Calcium supplements have been shown to reduce blood pressure in healthy people. We know that calcium channel blockers are hypotensive agents and they decrease calcium levels within the cells. It may be that calcium itself is a specific inhibitor of calcium channels *in vivo* (people) as it is *in vitro* (a controlled environment, such as a laboratory container).

Magnesium is regarded as nature's calcium channel blocker. It was first recommended for treatment of hypertension in the early 1900s. Magnesium is an important agent for lowering blood pressure, since magnesium deficiency within the cells is a major cause of hypertension. When dietary magnesium levels are high, blood pressure lowers. It is especially useful if you are on a diuretic when taking magnesium. One gram should be taken over the course of the day, along with 1.5 grams of calcium.

Essential fatty acids and ascorbic acid, or vitamin C, also have a role in the treatment of hypertension. Fish oils, especially omega 6 oils, reduce the blood vessels' response to hormones involved in hypertension. There are also studies that indicate that fish oils may facilitate

Sodium, Potassium, Calcium, and Phosphorus Content of Foods

FOOD	100 GRAMS	SODIUM (NA)	POTASSIUM (K)	NA/K	CALCIUM	PHOSPHORUS (P)	CA/P
Almonds, dried	80 nuts	7	800	0.01	220	490	0.45
Apple	1 medium	1	130	0.01	8	10	0.80
Avocado	½ medium	4	604	0.01	10	42	0.24
Bacon, cured, cooked	12 slices	990	240	4.12	12	190	0.06
Banana, raw	1 small	2	370	0.01	8	26	0.31
Beans, green, cooked	1 cup	6	180	0.03	60	45	1.33
Beans, white, cooked	½ cup	7	416	0.02	50	148	0.34
Beef, cooked	4 oz	60	335	0.18	13	7	1.86
Beef, hamburger	4 oz	50	400	0.12	12	175	0.07
Beets, red, canned	½ cup	230	150	1.53	18	17	1.06
Bread, white	4 slices	480	100	4.80	80	88	0.91
Bread, whole wheat	4 slices	480	252	1.90	100	208	0.48
Butter	20 tsp	150	3	50.00	3	3	1.00
Cabbage, raw	1 cup	17	195	0.09	50	20	2.50
Cantaloupe, raw	¼ melon	12	251	0.05	14	16	0.88
Carrots, raw	1 large	46	340	0.14	36	36	1.00
Cashews, raw	50 nuts	12	420	0.03	36	340	0.11
Cheese, cheddar	4 oz	800	100	8.00	480	520	0.92
Corn, canned	½ cup	216	90	2.40	50	3	16.67
Crackers, saltine	2 crackers	66	7	9.43	1	5	0.20
Cucumbers, raw	1 medium	8	160	0.05	16	20	0.80
Eggs, hard cooked	2 eggs	130	140	0.93	60	230	0.26
Fish sticks	4–5 sticks	180	390	0.46	11	167	0.07
Frankfurters, cooked	2 franks	950	190	5.00	4	100	0.04
Grapefruit, raw	½ medium	1	135	0.01	16	16	1.00
Halibut, broiled	3.5 oz	125	460	0.27	18	235	0.08
Lamb leg, roasted	3.5 oz	75	265	0.28	13	210	0.06
Lettuce, iceberg	1.5 cups	9	195	0.05	21	24	0.88

Food	Serving						
Liver	3.5 oz	165	355	0.46	12	450	0.03
Liverwurst	3.5 oz	270	220	1.23	10	220	0.05
Milk, whole	8 oz	122	351	0.35	288	227	1.27
Oatmeal, cooked	½ cup	250	65	3.85	10	65	0.15
Olives, green, canned	12 medium	1800	42	42.86	48	12	4.00
Onions, boiled	½ cup	7	120	0.06	24	30	0.80
Orange, raw	1 small	1	200	0.01	40	10	4.00
Orange juice	4 oz	1	220	0.00	10	18	0.56
Oysters, canned	3.5 oz	62	70	0.89	28	124	0.23
Peanut butter	4 oz	680	720	0.94	72	440	0.16
Peas, green	3.5 oz	230	95	2.42	26	70	0.37
Pickles, dill	1 medium	1500	210	7.14	27	21	1.29
Pineapple, raw	⅔ cup	1	165	0.01	20	8	2.50
Pork, lean, roasted	3.5 oz	1100	330	3.33	12	225	0.05
Potatoes, baked	1 medium	4	503	0.01	9	65	0.14
Raisins, raw	3.5 oz	30	700	0.04	60	95	0.63
Rice, brown, cooked	⅔ cup	265	65	4.08	12	70	0.17
Rice, white, cooked	⅔ cup	350	25	14.00	11	28	0.39
Salmon, baked	3.5 oz	120	410	0.29	75	380	0.20
Salt, table	1 tsp	388	0	****	3	2	1.50
Sardines, canned	3.5 oz	260	180	1.44	135	150	0.90
Shrimp, boiled	3.5 oz	115	185	0.62	70	195	0.36
Soybeans, boiled	⅔ cup	3	400	0.01	50	160	0.31
Spinach, raw	2 cups	80	500	0.16	100	56	1.79
Squash, boiled	½ cup		140	0.01	25	25	1.00
Sweet potato, baked	1 small	15	400	0.04	50	75	0.67
Tomato, raw	1 small	3	270	0.01	15	30	0.50
Tuna, canned	3.5 oz	700	260	2.69	8	240	0.03
Turkey, roasted	3.5 oz	85	400	0.21	10	280	0.04
Turnips, boiled	⅔ cup	36	190	0.19	35	24	1.46
Vegetables, mixed	⅔ cup	55	200	0.28	25	60	0.42
Walnuts, raw	30 nuts	0	420	0.00	60	350	0.17

COURTESY OF JOSEPH E. PIZZORNO, JR., N.D., BASTYR UNIVERSITY excretion of sodium and bodily fluids by the kidneys. Fish oils also increase urine output, resulting in a reduced fluid volume within the body. Take one 300–600 mg capsule per day.

Men with hypertension have low levels of vitamin C in their blood. A diet low in vitamin C is considered a dietary risk factor for high blood pressure. I recommend 1000 mg between two and four times a day, depending on the blood type.

GENERAL DIETARY SUGGESTIONS

Generally, people with hypertension consume higher amounts of salt than people who do not have hypertension. Once the body becomes accustomed to a diet high in salt, the taste threshold for salt increases, which means that the person eventually consumes larger amounts of salt to have the same taste. To make matters worse, the salt content of prepared, cured, smoked, or processed food has increased over the years. It is important to read the labels of commercial foods. You should watch out for other forms of salt, including sodium chloride, MSG, monosodium, and Na (the chemical symbol for salt). Foods high in sodium include items like teriyaki or soy sauce, baking powder, and some antacids. Ideally, stay away from processed foods. And beware of "salt substitutes," which can be made of up to 50 percent sodium chloride. Vegetarians generally have lower blood pressures, not necessarily because their intake of sodium is different but because their intake of potassium, fiber, calcium, magnesium, complex carbohydrates, essential fatty acids, and vitamins A and C are more commonly found in a vegetarian diet.

It is extremely important if you're suffering from hypertension to eat according to your blood type. Be sure to consume a diet high in whole, unprocessed foods like whole grains, legumes, vegetables, fruits, nuts, and seeds. If you are blood type B or O, you should also consume animal protein in the form of an occasional piece of lean, chemical-free lamb and veal, turkey, chicken (for blood type O only), and the cold-water, top fish mentioned earlier. Caffeine, alcohol, tobacco, and sugar should be avoided completely.

Caffeine, which can be found in large doses in items like chocolate, sodas, and coffee, will consistently increase blood pressure for several days after consumption—regardless of one's hypertensive condition. Usually the blood pressure reaches its normal state after a few days, but only if you stop drinking these beverages on a regular basis. The body doesn't have time to reach its normal blood pressure if you drink coffee daily.

Alcohol, when consumed regularly, is one of the greatest contributors to high blood pressure. Acute hypertension can be produced in some people who drink only moderate amounts of alcohol.

Many of us know that smoking also contributes to hypertension. But don't forget that snuff, chewing tobacco, and any other form of smokeless tobacco can cause hypertension because of their nicotine and sodium content. People who smoke also usually have increased consumption of sugar, alcohol, and caffeine. Compared to nonsmokers, cigarette smokers have higher levels of lead (which is elevated in a significant number of hypertensive males) and cadmium (known to contribute to hypertension) while having lower levels of ascorbic acid.

EXERCISE AND STRESS REDUCTION

Exercise is just as important as herbs and nutrients in the treatment of hypertension. Studies have shown a 35–52 percent increased risk for hypertension in people who are sedentary. Regular exercise creates a sustained decrease in systolic and diastolic blood pressure. It is crucial to participate in the type of exercise specified for your blood type. As discussed in Chapter Four, "Nutrition and Your Blood Type," those with types O and B should do an aerobic exercise, while those with types A and AB should engage in a gentler type of exercise, like yoga or tai chi. Hypertensive type As and ABs should do some form of aerobic exercise, but nothing too strenuous. I advise patients to do race walking or low-impact aerobics. Generally, all blood types will gain great benefits from at least one or two relaxation techniques such as yoga, biofeedback, meditation, or progressive muscle relaxation.

7

DIABETES

A CASE

Last year an African-American gentleman came into my office for his initial visit. Before I could even ask my first question, he began talking. "I have diabetes and a touch of arthritis," he said. "I've been angry a lot lately—I used to repress it but it's gotten worse lately. I let people know how angry I am and lots of times I withdraw from things." As he told me these things, I noticed how rigid he was. Every muscle in his body seemed to be tensed.

Darrell continued by telling me that until three years ago he and his wife thought they could find reconciliation in their troubled marriage. But then around that time she got pregnant. And he was *not* the father.

Together they had had a boy, and though his wife wanted him to spend more time with the kid, she didn't make it easy to visit the child. "Every time I go to visit him she looks at me as if I crawled out of the sewer," he said. The new man in her life asked that Darrell not come by the house so often. Darrell said he had recently had an argument with her over the phone and hung up on her. "I wanted to bash her face in," he said.

At first, when things started to get bad, he really wanted to work things out. "I have a story in my head about being in a good relationship. My parents separated when I was a child; my mom left my dad because he had a girlfriend. When I was ten, his bad habit killed him—his girlfriend shot him dead."

Darrell was in college when he first noticed the signs of diabetes. He was in his first marriage and raising a child who had brain damage.

"My son died when he was thirteen," he said, weeping. "I miss him so. I was so hurt and disappointed." His weeping turned into heavy sobbing as he continued: "I had my life planned—marriage, the military. I had direction, and all of a sudden my life was changed by my son's death and my diabetes." Because of his diagnosis, he was given a medical discharge the day before he was to be commissioned. He felt frightened and hopeless.

As a child, he and his mother lived with his grandparents after his dad died. He loved his grandmother dearly, but on the day of his twelfth birthday his grandmother died. His mother, who had never shown much affection, had a new boyfriend who did not care for him, so Darrell was sent to live with his aunt and uncle.

Darrell was a weakling as a child. He was seldom chosen for any team sport and was frequently teased and humiliated. Now he confessed to being opinionated, intolerant, inflexible and private. He told me he drove dangerously fast and had accumulated speeding tickets from state to state. He also said he had fantasies about shooting or beating up an authority figure. He even imagined carrying a weapon in order to give him an inflated sense of power. In addition to violent fantasies, he said, he had sexual fantasies and masturbated three to four times a week.

Given these circumstances, it was no surprise to hear he overreacted to the slightest offense, sometimes even imagined offenses. While his fear of strangers had lessened, his confidence among other people was still extremely low. His memory and concentration also were very poor. In addition to the diabetes, he complained of excessive flatulence, abdominal bloating, and joint pains.

I understood that this patient had been taunted as a child because of his inability to perform in ways that promote confidence, especially in younger boys. Without the affection and attention of his mother, or the guidance of his father, he had little or no support or encouragement from anyone who cared. His confidence back then was minimal at best. The resulting emotion was anger. When the only person who seemed to care about him—his grandmother—died, he decided God was to blame. His anger deepened.

Now as an adult, after losing a son, a wife and a planned life with direction and support, his anger continued to fester and his bitterness was manifesting itself in violent fantasies. The violence seemed to be a substitute for his lack of confidence. For this combination of inferiority and cruelty, I prescribed the homeopathic remedy anacardium 200 c.

When the herb anacardium is given to a healthy person, it creates a feeling of anxiety and uneasiness. The person experiences sadness because of feelings of inadequacy. Sometimes the person will also believe that harm will come to him. Slight offenses create irritability and anger—to the point of violence and violent fantasies. Memory gets weaker and concentration becomes more difficult. Physical symptoms can include headaches, vertigo, arthritis, gastritis, ulcer, and can also include diabetes. It is clear how anacardium's symptoms made it the logical choice to prescribe for Darrell.

WHAT IS DIABETES?

It is estimated that over 16 million Americans (4.5 percent of the population) have diabetes, but only a little over half of the people actually know they have it. We consider a person to be diabetic when exhibiting the following clinical picture:

- ❦ A fasting (overnight) blood glucose (sugar) level is greater than or equal to 140 mg/dl on at least two separate occasions; and
- ❦ A blood glucose level is greater than or equal to 200 mg/dl two hours after ingestion (the end of the testing period) of 75 g of glucose and a similar result for one other sample during the two-hour testing period.

Clinical symptoms of diabetes include excessive and frequent urination and thirst, with excessive appetite and weight loss. Because these symptoms are not life-threatening, many people with diabetes do not seek medical care.

Diabetes rates are 60 percent higher among African-Americans than among white Americans. Interestingly, diabetes was not a problem for us until the beginning of the twentieth century. Africans are not predisposed to diabetes and African slaves did not come to America with diabetes. This bears witness to what we know in naturopathy: that people begin to acquire harmful diseases like diabetes when they begin to indulge in Western diets and lifestyles.

Often called "sugar diabetes," diabetes mellitus is a disorder of the body's ability to utilize sugar, or glucose, resulting in fasting elevations of blood sugar levels. Fat and protein metabolism are also disrupted, resulting in increased risk of heart disease, stroke, kidney disease, and loss of nerve and sexual function.

Before our bodies can use food as fuel, it must be converted into glucose. The glucose enters the cells and is used for energy so the cells can function. Insulin, a hormone manufactured by the islets cells of the pancreas, is essential for glucose to enter the cells. In a nondiabetic person, rising blood glucose levels trigger the pancreas to secrete insulin. Insulin attaches to glucose and carries it into the millions of cells in the body. When glucose levels decrease, however, the liver releases its stored form of glucose so that the blood sugar levels can rise again. If, as in the case of a diabetic person, the pancreas does not secrete enough insulin, or if the cells become resistant to insulin, the blood sugar cannot get into the cells, and the cells starve as glucose increases in the blood. To make matters worse, low insulin levels make the body think that it needs glucose. In response, the liver pours more glucose into the blood.

The symptoms of diabetes—excessive urination, thirst, appetite, and weight loss—are the result of the body's attempt to rid itself of the glucose in the blood and use it for energy. High blood sugar levels, for example, stimulate the kidneys to excrete large amounts of urine because it contains glucose. The high level of sugar in the blood also makes the blood thicker in concentration. So in addition to the loss of water through urination, the diabetic person's thirst increases with the thickness of the blood. Weight loss results from cells that starve because they lack nourishing glucose. The patient may eat excessive amounts of food to combat this problem, but the glucose in the food passes through and is lost in the urine.

Two Types of Diabetes

There are two types of diabetes: Type I and Type II. Resulting from a lack of insulin in the body, Type I is called insulin-dependent diabetes mellitus (IDDM). IDDM occurs most often in children and adolescents, which is why this condition is often called "juvenile diabetes." IDDM means there is complete destruction of the beta cells of the pancreas, where insulin is made. Approximately 10 percent of all diabetics are Type I. The exact cause is unknown, but it is believed to be the result of injury to the beta cells and a defect in tissue regeneration. In a majority of Type I cases, the patient usually has a high number of beta-cell antibodies. It is likely that the antibodies to the beta cells develop as a result of cell destruction by free radicals, a virus, food allergies, or chemicals such as pesticides found in agriculture and those used to smoke and cure meats. Recent research indicates that early exposure in infancy to a protein in cow's milk may be an important determinant of Type I diabetes, specifically increasing the risk by 1.5 times. *Type I diabetics will almost always require some insulin, but the amount can be reduced using the principles of naturopathy and the suggestions discussed in this chapter.* **[Note: If you are insulin dependent, do not stop your insulin under any circumstances unless instructed by a physician.]**

With Type II diabetics, insulin production is not the central problem. The problem is the body's inability to use insulin effectively. For some reason, the cells are not sensitive enough to insulin, and therefore do not properly utilize glucose. Occurring in people middle-aged or older, this type of diabetes is often called "adult onset," but is otherwise known as non-insulin-dependent diabetes mellitus (NIDDM). The symptoms listed above may or may not be experienced by the person with Type II diabetes. But there are other symptoms, such as fatigue, blurred vision, frequent infections, or wounds that are slow to heal. Ninety percent of those who have diabetes have this type. It is usually discovered during a routine examination. In many cases the patient is overweight or obese, inactive, and over the age of forty.

The major contributing factor for insulin insensitivity and the onset of diabetes is poor diet. I repeatedly remind my patients that you cannot "catch" diabetes (or hypertension for that matter) from other people. We become more susceptible because of the toxins in our bodies that have accumulated from unhealthy lifestyles and diets. And people who have family members with diabetes or who are African-American, Native American, or Hispanic are at greater risk statistically for developing diabetes. Our diets, which are usually high in sugar, fats, and animal products, only aid in our susceptibility to this disease. Refined carbohydrates are among the most important contributing factors to the diabetic condition (and also to obesity). Sugars are quickly absorbed into the bloodstream, causing a rapid rise in blood sugar. And a diet high in fat increases the risks for NIDDM. Approximately 80 percent of people with NIDDM are overweight. Obesity, or body fat percentage greater than 25 to 30 percent, is also highly associated with insulin insensitivity. Lack of exercise and vitamin and mineral deficiency contribute as well.

DIABETIC COMPLICATIONS

People who suffer from diabetes are often victims of other medical complications, such as atherosclerosis, diabetic neuropathy, diabetic retinopathy, diabetic nephropathy, and diabetic foot ulcers. The diabetic patient has two or three times as great a risk of dying from atherosclerosis (a hardening of the arteries due to cholesterol buildup) as the nondiabetic person. It is therefore essential to lower cholesterol levels through change of diet and lifestyle. For example, the person must eat less saturated fat by reducing animal products, increase the amount of fiber intake from plants (vegetables, grains, legumes), and exercise more. One should also eliminate smoking and coffee (both decaffeinated and caffeinated) to help prevent athlerosclerosis.

Tingling sensations, numbness, loss of peripheral nerve function, pain, and muscle weakness are signs of diabetic neuropathies. The neuropathies (any disease of the nervous system that is not in the brain or spinal cord) typically occur on both sides of the body. Diabetics with neuropathy have been found to be deficient in vitamin B6, as will be discussed later in this chapter.

Retinopathy, another complication from diabetes, is the leading cause of blindness in the United States. One in twenty Type I diabetics and one in fifteen Type II diabetics develop retinopathy. Hemorrhages, swelling, or detachment of the innermost lining of the back of the eyeball can occur, and are forms of retinopathic lesions or areas of disease or injury to the retina of the eye—that part of the eye that receives images produced by the lens. Vitamin C has been shown to be effective with conditions of the eye, because it reduces sorbitol, a byproduct of glucose. (In nondiabetics, sorbitol metabolizes into fructose and is ultimately excreted by the cell. In a diabetic, however, the sorbitol accumulates and plays a significant role in the chronic complications of diabetes.)

Another common complication of diabetes involves the kidneys. There are several ways the kidney may be compromised, but the most likely is when the filter for the blood's impurities hardens. The result is usually hypertension, edema (swelling of the limbs), and protein in the urine (proteinuria). Unless something is done, the kidney simply fails.

If the blood supply to the limbs or any part of the body is constricted, an ischemic condition (see Glossary) may arise. Ischemia, along with peripheral neuropathy, is the main cause of diabetic foot ulcers.

But foot ulcers and gangrene are preventable. Proper foot care is essential. You must keep your feet clean, dry, and warm. Wear shoes that fit comfortably and, of course, avoid injury to the foot. Smoking or the use of tobacco products can cause vasoconstriction (constriction of the blood vessels) of the lower limbs. Massage and hydrotherapy (the application of hot or cold water to various parts of the body to produce a specific effect) can help increase circulation. Massage should be gentle and in an upward motion, toward the heart. Hot compresses can be applied to the lower abdomen and groin area to increase circulation in the lower limbs. *Do not apply heat directly to the lower limbs if you have peripheral neuropathy or loss of circulation.* Also do not compromise the circulation by sitting with your legs crossed or up under your buttocks.

CASE II

John, a Caucasian male, came to my office because his blood sugar was rising despite the medication he had been taking. He had been diabetic and overweight for over ten years and was now more concerned because he was losing the sensation in his toes (a sign of peripheral neuropathy). He came to me because he wanted change in his life, change in "the deep-seated patterns and ways of thinking about himself."

He told me the following story. Though born in the United States, he had spent some of his childhood outside of this country. When his parents moved back to the United States he did not feel as though this was his country. "I was miserable. Anyone with a foreign accent was not all right. I had a difficult time with English. I had no friends, because I didn't like most of the people I met and they didn't like me. I felt angry a lot of the time." His parents sent him back out of the country to live with relatives. "I was happy to be back in my place, so I would not feel this out-of-place misery."

Because he was so unhappy as a child he had great empathy for "an unhappy society," which is where he spent his junior high, high school, and college years. The country in which he lived was involved in war at the time and he was on the side of the people. "I was outraged and wanted to help. It felt like an undoing of what I lived through as a child. I felt I could make life better for people. The government had enriched itself, shamefully."

John was in a relationship for two years with a woman with whom he had a son. As she and her son were delivering supplies to another town military troops shot and killed them. It was later reported that they killed "dangerous guerrillas." "That was part of the life there." He weeps and says, "But a nine-month-old is not dangerous, Dr. Sullivan." He left the county several months later. "I had so much grief that had nowhere to go, so I worked harder and longer. It was a way to deal with the pain. My body has run out of steam. My body does not want to work seventy to eighty hours a week. I have a temper. I can be short, nasty, and mean. I can feel overwhelmed and ask myself, 'Why all these demands and burdens, why me?' Life is too much, I can't stand it—the lack of time, money, and so many demands. I stew on it and turn inward; occasionally I shout but not often. I am exploding inside."

John is a very compassionate and kind man, deeply affected by the state of the world. "I see people with no support in their lives, no resources; their lives are impossible. It's so wrong and unfair that I want to just scream about it some days. Sometimes I am not thinking. I am wounded and confused. The injustice in this country is so cruel."

John's intense empathy and willingness to stand up and participate against a system that suppresses the lives and hopes of people less fortunate than himself was sparked by his own painful childhood. He knew firsthand what it was like to feel as though he was strange, different, unwanted and inferior. His grief about and outrage at the injustice in this world, coupled with the murder of his girlfriend and his son, were responsible for creating the susceptibility to diabetes. His father was also diabetic, but that does not mean that John would have been necessarily. Without these tragedies and with proper nutrition, I believe John could have maintained a normal blood sugar. I gave John the remedy causticum in a 200 c potency for the dis-ease he felt owing to the intense sympathy for the people in the world, his personal grief, and for his body, which manifested diabetes.

While much of John's diet was fruits, vegetables and whole grains, he did make a habit of eating too many white flour products and very little animal protein. After he was placed on a modified detox diet (that included fish) and received colonics, I gave him a diet for his blood type and added some of the herbs that you will read about in subsequent sections of this chapter.

Four months after John's initial visit he reported more sensation in his feet and hands. "My feet and I are feeling less dead. I am feeling more energy. My voice is louder. My blood sugar has been in the 100's. It has not been in the 200's since I first came here. I feel like Spirit has created a space for me to be in and it's safe. I am aware I am doing things differently in my life. It's easier to say no to people. I make time to do other things besides work."

While John's blood sugar continues to decrease, his treatment is ongoing as he must be mindful to eat well most of the time. It may take as long as two or three years to normalize John's blood sugar and the sensations in his feet and hands, but the improvement is consistent. Natural medicine takes time because it is healing a system, not suppressing an organ or replacing its function. The herbs and supplements I prescribed for John are discussed in detail below.

HERBAL TREATMENTS AND NUTRITIONAL SUPPLEMENTS

As you know now, many diseases were treated with plants and minerals before the advent of synthetic drugs. Diabetes is no different. Before insulin, we used plants to manage this disease. And there is much research detailing the efficacy of plants on diabetes. I have outlined below the ones used in my practice.

- ❧ Bitter melon, or *Mormordica charantia,* is a tropical fruit cultivated in Africa and Asia. It looks like an unattractive cucumber because of its bumpy covering. The fresh juice or the extract of the unripe fruit has hypoglycemic properties (it lowers blood sugar). As the name suggests, this fruit is a bitter substance that is unpleasant in taste. While it could be put in water to reduce the harsh taste, simply drinking 2 ounces of fresh juice, three times a day, is the most effective approach. Bitter melon can be found at Asian grocery stores. Health food stores have tinctures and extracts that are not quite as effective as the fresh juice but can be used in the same dosage.

❧ Garlic, or *Allium sativum,* and onions, or *Allium cepa,* have sulfur-containing compounds that help to regulate blood sugar and increase serum insulin. When these plants are eaten, the sulfur-containing portions of the plants compete with insulin (which also contains sulfur) in the liver. More free insulin then becomes available in the blood. I usually prescribe ½ clove of garlic two times a day (or 2 garlic capsules, totaling 800 to 1000 mg), and 1–7 ounces of onion (raw or boiled), along with the herb fenugreek.

❧ *Trigonella foenumgraecum* or fenugreek seeds have antidiabetic properties. They reduce fasting and postprandial blood glucose levels, as well as total cholesterol and triglycerides, while increasing HDL-cholesterol ("good" cholesterol). Studies have shown that, when 50 grams were administered twice daily to diabetics on insulin, there were significant reductions in blood sugar and an improved glucose tolerance.

❧ *Gymnema sylvestre* is another herb proven effective in the treatment of both types of diabetes. Several years ago manufacturers claimed that this herb could block the absorption of sugar. This is not true. Gymnema does block the sensation of sweetness, but it does not block the absorption of sugar. Gymnema also increases the production of endogenous insulin, regenerates insulin-producing beta cells in the pancreas, reduces insulin requirements and fasting blood sugar levels. The recommended dosage is 400 mg per day.

❧ Plants that contain a compound, flavonoid, called epicatechin, may also be useful in the treatment of diabetics because of their antioxidant properties. It has been demonstrated that these flavonoids prevent damage of beta cells in diabetic animals. They also aid in the regeneration of these cells. The most common source of the epicatechin compound is the plant *Camellia chinensis,* or green tea. You should take two four-ounce cups a day.

❧ Bilberry leaf tea (European blueberry or *Vaccinium myrtillus*) has a long history of use for diabetics. One of the compounds, myrtillin (an anthocyanoside), in the plant acts like insulin. There is also an increase in vitamin C in the cells and a decrease in the leakage and breakage of small blood vessels. In particular, bilberry leaf helps the vessels of the eye and the retina, and is valuable in treating diabetic retinopathy, cataracts, and night blindness. The dosage is 80 to 160 mg, three times a day.

❧ *Ginkgo biloba* extract is known for its ability to increase blood flow to the brain, which helps improve one's memory. But it also increases blood flow to the arms, fingers, legs and toes. I recommend 40 mg, three times a day.

As I said in the preceding chapters, everyone should take a good multiple vitamin on a regular basis, simply to combat the poor quality of some of our foods, the stress of life and the pollutants in our environment. You should be sure, however, to take some supplements if you are diabetic, especially chromium, vitamin C and B complex. In 1854 brewer's yeast was found to have a positive effect on diabetes. This is because brewer's yeast contains chromium and amino acids. Chromium works with insulin in facilitating the intake of glucose into the cells. Some studies have found that supplementing the diet with chromium has decreased fasting glucose levels, improved glucose tolerance, lowered insulin levels, and reduced total cholesterol. Other studies have not supported the finding that chromium improves glucose tolerance, but it has been shown to be essential in blood sugar metabolism. Because of this and the fact that chromium deficiency is common owing to agricultural methods that rob foods of vital minerals, I prescribe 400 mcg per day, preferably in the picolinate form.

Vitamin C is another important supplement for diabetes. For example, 2000 mg a day of vitamin C will reduce the accumulation of sorbitol in the red blood cells of diabetics and inhibit one of the biochemical processes that leads to complications of the eyes and nerves. Vitamin C also helps with other complications, like excessive bruising, slow healing, bleeding gums, and susceptibility to infection. The reason is that vitamin C is important in the manufacture of collagen, the primary protein substance in the body. For those with adult onset diabetes, vitamin C has been found to decrease fasting blood insulin levels and total cholesterol. I suggest 1000 mg, two to four times a day.

Vitamin B complex is another supplement I prescribe because of its role in energy production and fat, cholesterol, and carbohydrate metabolism. The enzymes that play a vital role in these bodily functions need niacin (vitamin B3). Niacin also plays a role in glucose tolerance. Niacinamide, a form of niacin (or nicotinic acid), has been used in several studies that have found the importance of niacin in the prevention of Type I diabetes. It has also been used to regenerate the beta cells or slow their destruction. There is evidence from these studies that niacin can prolong the periods of time when diabetics are not in need of daily doses of insulin. It can also possibly lower insulin requirements and increase beta-cell function. The doses depend on body weight, 25 mg per kilogram. Generally, I prescribe 100 to 200 mg per day.

Another form of niacin is inositol hexaniacinate, which can also be used in Type I and Type II diabetes, especially for the lowering of blood fats. You may know of niacin creating a flushing of the skin and gastric irritation when taken in high doses (3 grams). There are "time-released" products that cause less immediate reaction but are ultimately more toxic to the liver. Inositol is not only gentler on the liver but also gives better results with blood sugar regulation. Used in Europe to reduce blood cholesterol and increase the blood flow to the lower extremities, inositol can be found in any good B complex vitamin, taken in standard doses.

Other vitamins in a B complex will include biotin and B6. Biotin is involved in the making and using of carbohydrates, fats, and amino acids. Biotin is made in the intestines by intestinal bacteria. It has been shown to increase insulin sensitivity and the activity of the enzyme that is responsible for the first step in the liver's use of glucose. Vitamin B6 is essential for any diabetic to prevent or treat diabetic neuropathy. It is also important to have adequate levels of B6 in order to facilitate the cellular intake of magnesium. The amount prescribed is typically 150 mg per day.

Minerals such as magnesium, potassium, manganese, and zinc

should also be a part of diabetic supplements. These minerals will most likely be included in your multivitamin. It is necessary to supplement them because diabetic patients not only need more of these minerals but often lose valuable amounts in their urine. Some diabetics are on medication for high blood pressure such as diuretics, which also waste minerals. Magnesium plays a role in carbohydrate metabolism and insulin activity. Magnesium levels are lowest in those diabetics with severe retinopathy, which suggests that mineral supplements may be helpful. Though magnesium is found in our foods, food processing strips foods of this nutrient. I recommend 300 to 500 mg of magnesium aspartate or citrate.

Potassium is another essential mineral, but people with diabetes or kidney disease have difficulty handling excessive amounts of potassium. It is best to get this mineral in the form of vegetable juices (beets, carrots, celery, or a combination of kale, collards, and seaweed). Potassium improves insulin sensitivity and secretion and reduces the risk of heart disease, atherosclerosis and cancer.

Manganese can be found in many enzyme systems that are responsible for blood sugar control and energy metabolism. In animals, a deficiency of manganese results in diabetes. Diabetics have only half as much manganese as nondiabetics. Recommended dosage is 30 mg per day.

The last mineral for review is zinc, which is essential in making, releasing, and using insulin. It also helps prevent beta-cell destruction. As with other minerals, zinc is excreted in large amounts in the urine of diabetics. Wounds that are slow to heal are also aided by zinc supplementation. I prescribe 30 to 50 mg per day.

Two other important nutrients are flavonoids and essential fatty acids. Flavonoids are plant pigments that make carrots and sweet potatoes orange, blueberries blue, and cherries dark red. As will be discussed in Chapter 9, "Arthritis," flavonoids perform a myriad of functions. They reduce inflammation and slow down the production of prostaglandins. They increase the absorption of vitamin C, neutralize free radicals, and strengthen capillaries. They also protect healthy cells by stabilizing the inflammatory cell membrane, thereby reducing the release of histamine. Flavonoids have antiallergic, antiviral, and anticarcinogenic properties. Type I diabetics should increase their intake of flavonoids to guard against damage to beta cells and to promote insulin secretion.

But because flavonoids also help inhibit the accumulation of sorbitol, which creates complications of the eyes, all diabetics should consider increasing their intake. One to two grams of mixed flavonoids is recommended.

Essential fatty acids are a necessary part of the diet of diabetics. GLA, or gamma linolenic acid, is an essential fatty acid (or omega 6 fatty acid) that protects against diabetic neuropathy. A disturbance in essential fatty acid metabolism can lead to reduced blood flow and oxygen to neurons (the cells of the nervous system). Sources of GLA include borage, black currant oil, or evening primrose oil, as well as many nuts and seeds and their oils—sunflower, safflower, pecans, sesame, and Brazil. Supplementing the diet with 450 mg a day is sufficient.

Omega 3 fatty acid oils, or alpha linolenic acid, guards against atherosclerosis and increases insulin secretion in diabetics who are non–insulin dependent. Flaxseed oil—one tablespoon daily—is a good source of omega 3 oils. Cold-water fish, such as salmon, halibut, mackerel, and herring, are also excellent sources of this fatty acid. There are studies that indicate that cultures that eat these fish regularly have a much lower incidence of both types of diabetes. Three- to four-ounce servings, two times per week, are adequate.

As I mentioned earlier, diet is the most important factor in the prevention and treatment of diabetes. Aside from the diets based on blood types, there are other guidelines a diabetic needs to follow to minimize the risk of complications and have a high quality of life.

GENERAL DIETARY SUGGESTIONS

There is considerable evidence indicating the Western diet and lifestyle as the causative factors in the development of diabetes. If you are diabetic, you *must* avoid certain foods. Specifically, you need to remove all refined and processed sugars, carbohydrates, and fats from your diet. Say goodbye to cakes, pies, and cookies made with white flour, white sugar and butter. Replace them, if you must, with pastries that are made with whole grains (spelt, whole wheat, kamut, and other unbleached flours) and use fruit juice, maple syrup, or succanat as a sweetener. Fruits are much better than white flour or white sugar when it comes to regulating blood sugar levels.

Just as you must eliminate consumption of white flour and white sugar, you must add fiber to your diet, because diabetes has been linked with inadequate dietary fiber. As discussed in Chapter 4, "Nutrition and Your Blood Type," water-soluble fiber slows down digestion and absorption of carbohydrates, thus preventing a rapid increase of blood sugar. It helps prevent the excessive secretion of insulin and increases the liver's uptake of glucose. Water-soluble fiber can be found primarily in most vegetables, oat bran, beans, pears, apples, nuts, seeds, and psyllium seed husks (edible seeds from the plantain). Supplementing this with preparations of plant fibers like guar gum and pectin is also effective at dosages of 5 grams and 10 grams per meal, respectively. Please note, however, that this supplementation is not intended to substitute for a high-fiber diet.

Generally, your diet should be very similar to the detoxification diet on p. 69. This diet is high in grains, beans and legumes, and vegetables, which are all high in fiber. Though protein is restricted on the detoxification diet, diabetics should consume small amounts. Basically a diet that is high in *complex* carbohydrates, low in protein and fat is what I prescribe for all diabetics.

But don't forget that your blood type is still important. For example, the patient at the beginning of this chapter is a blood type O. Darrell was advised to eat complex carbohydrates, especially cereals like kamut, amaranth, millet, spelt, puffed rice, and kasha. Because whole wheat will create bloating and digestive problems for a blood type O, I asked him to eat sprouted whole wheat (Ezekiel or Essene), multigrains (like kamut, spelt, oats, or millet) or millet breads.

Blood type O's have a wide variety of vegetables and legumes available to them. I instructed Darrell to eat plenty of broccoli, escarole, beet and dandelion leaves, kale and collard greens (without the pork), Swiss chard, parsnips, onions, garlic, okra, pumpkin and butternut squash, turnips, red peppers, spinach, and seaweed. Asparagus, carrots, cucumbers, lettuce, watercress, and radishes were also permitted, but only in moderation. I encouraged him to eat dried beans like black-eyed peas, pinto, azuki, and garbanzo (chick peas) at least two or three times per week.

I told Darrell to eat fruits sometimes instead of breads and pasta. They are not only a good source of fiber, but they also help with the weight control of most diabetics. Fruits for blood type O's need to be more alkaline (as opposed to acidic fruits like oranges and strawberries). Plums, prunes, and figs should be eaten regularly. Grapefruit is another good option, because it becomes alkaline when it is digested. Blueberries, bananas, pears, grapes, apples, peaches, cherries, papaya, and raisins may also be eaten in moderation. As much as possible, these fruits (and vegetables, too) should be organic and eaten separately from other foods.

Darrell learned that he could eat very lean, chemical-free meat, such as veal and lamb, three to five times per week. And I told him to eat fish—salmon, halibut, herring, snapper, mackerel, sardine, rainbow trout, and striped bass—baked or broiled, three times a week, in five- to six-ounce portions. I suggested he eat free-range, chemical-free chicken and turkey, but only one or two times a week. Keeping in mind the principles of proper food combining, I asked him to eat animal protein only with vegetables, not with complex carbohydrates.

Even a diabetic who is blood type A needs to eat some animal protein. For these people, I recommend poultry and seafood (not shellfish; preferably salmon, rainbow trout, sardine, monkfish, grouper, and perch) two to three times per week each, in five-ounce servings. Mindful of the health of their kidneys, I make sure they drink lots of water and tea (like *buchu* and *solidago*). Blood type A's should not consume whole milk products, because they are poorly digested and stimulate insulin reactions. As indicated in the detox diet, soy is an excellent substitute for dairy products.

EXERCISE

Exercise increases our cells' sensitivity to insulin and the biological effects of insulin. When we exercise, our muscles remove glucose from the blood more efficiently than when we are at rest. It is important to follow the recommended exercises for your blood type (see Chapter 4, "Nutrition and Your Blood Type"). Even blood type A's, however, need some aerobic exercise if they are diabetic. If you are Type II diabetic, you should do some low-intensity aerobics, like brisk walking, at least five times per week for forty-five minutes to an hour. Of course, blood type O's and B's will need some more strenuous exercise.

If you are Type I diabetic, your exercise should be carefully monitored along with your insulin and carbohydrate consumption. You should increase the dosage of insulin or increase the carbohydrate consumption prior to exercise, being mindful to inject part of the body that will not be active during exercise. It is beneficial to eat a carbohydrate before and during prolonged exercise. And do not exercise during peak insulin times. If you have retinopathy, swimming would be better for you than exercise that bounces you up and down.

Three months into the treatment, Darrell's mental and emotional state had improved. "I feel like I'm standing in sunshine, not cold clouds," he said. "I'm definitely not as angry, my solitude is pleasant. My arthritis is gone."

During his next visit he said to me, "My anger is rarely an issue anymore. When I find something to be angry about, I deal with it and rarely fantasize. My confidence is pretty good these days. Now I'm thinking there's no such thing as a stranger. I walked up to a woman today who looked nice. Not that I was attracted to her, but I just wanted to say, 'Hi.' I just wanted to make friends." Though still dependent on insulin, Darrell's blood sugar levels had lowered and were more consistent.

Diabetic patients do not always have such great responses in such a brief period of time. Sometimes the process is longer and the results may not come as dramatically and quickly. Natural medicine takes time because the goal is to heal, not to suppress. But diabetes is a manageable condition and natural therapies can be used effectively to change the course of the disease.

8

OBESITY

While studying in Greece in 1995, I happened to have lunch one day with an English couple who had recently returned from visiting their daughter in the southeastern part of the United States. During our conversation, I asked what impressed them the most about America. The man replied, "The number of Baptist churches and obese people!" I thought, of all the beautiful things in this country, how interesting and unfortunate it was that he was so taken by overweight Americans.

But how could he not be taken when one considers that 20 to 50 percent of Americans are obese? We know that physical inactivity and poor diet together account for at least 300,000 deaths in the United States each year—only tobacco use contributes to more preventable deaths. From the seventies to the nineties, obesity has increased by 54 percent among children ages six to eleven, and 39 percent among adolescents ages twelve to seventeen. Eighty percent of all obese teenagers are likely to become obese adults. Twenty-seven percent of adult women are obese, but that figure jumps to 45 to 50 percent for all black women!

Thirty-five to 65 percent of the United States adult population is "overweight," a term that must be distinguished from obesity. Being overweight refers to having an excess of body weight relative to body height. A person who is obese is always overweight, but not vice versa. Twenty-two percent of adolescent females and 20 percent of adolescent males were overweight in the early nineties. Donna Shalala, the Secretary of Health and Human services at the time of this survey, said, "It is clear that too many of our teenagers are overweight because they are inactive." Shalala went on to quote figures from the Centers for Disease Control, which reported that only 37 percent of ninth through twelfth graders engaged in at least twenty minutes of vigorous exercise at least three times a week, while 35 percent of them watched at least three hours of TV a day.

The word "obesity" applies to people who have an excess amount of body fat, 30 percent for women and 20–25 percent for men. Official measurements for obesity are determined by height and weight indices of life insurance companies. These companies rate men and women under three separate body frames: small, medium, and large. But these indices have received much criticism because they are based on the weight of people who have the lowest mortality rates among insured individuals. Also, the weight ranges for the lowest mortality rates do not necessarily reflect optimal weight for their height. For example, smokers are included in these surveys even though they do not always fall into a healthy weight range. In fact, a lot of smokers are underweight. It is also possible for someone to have excess body fat and still fall within a proper weight range. But suffice it to say, weight alone is a poor determinant of obesity. Most people who are overweight or obese know they are without the use of tables or measurements.

TYPES OF OBESITY

Obesity may be the result of excessive food intake and/or a low metabolic rate. Types of obesity are based on the size and number of adipose (fat) cells. *Hyperplastic* obesity occurs when fat cells increase in number and *hypertrophic* obesity occurs when the fat cells increase in size. The former usually develops in childhood and is not closely associated with metabolic dysfunction. In normal-weight infants, fat cell size increases slightly, but fat cell size triples or quadruples between birth and age two. Between age two and puberty, the number of fat cells is fairly constant. But for obese children, fat cell count increases along with fat cell size. Hypertrophic obesity, meanwhile, is more likely associated with metabolic problems. It tends to be associated with diabetes, hypertension, and hyperlipidemia (high cholesterol and triglycerides).

There is also a classification of obesity based on fat distribution. *Android* obesity involves fat deposited primarily in the upper body, such as the abdomen. *Gynecoid* obesity involves fat deposited in the lower body, such as the buttocks and thighs.

Specific types of obesity are associated with certain medical conditions. The incidence of diabetes mellitus, for instance, is higher in both men and women with hypertrophic, android obesity. Hypertension and hyperglycemia (high blood sugar, but not quite diabetes) are linked with android obesity. And as a part of treating certain medical conditions like arthritis, diabetes, and hypertension, it is essential to treat the person's obesity, regardless of classification.

Obesity increases the risk of illness and death due to diabetes, stroke, coronary artery disease, respiratory dysfunction, and kidney and gall bladder disease. Obesity is also closely associated with an increased incidence of some types of cancer, like endometrial. And generally, obesity decreases the ability of the body to produce antibodies that guard against disease and decreases the ability of the white blood cells to kill bacteria.

Complications of Obesity

Obesity can have devastating psychological effects on an individual. I will discuss those effects later in the chapter. Other complications include those of mechanical, metabolic, cardiovascular, respiratory, and dermatological (skin) nature, It can also significantly shorten life expectancy. An increase of twenty-five pounds above the standard weight range reduces life expectancy for a middle-aged person by nearly 25 percent.

Our bodies were not designed to work efficiently with substantial excess weight. Thus, obese people suffer commonly from osteoarthritis of the knees, hips, and lower back. And because the heart has to work harder to circulate blood in larger bodies, high blood pressure is more common among obese people, as are hypertension, diabetes mellitus, and cholesterol stones in the gall bladder. In more serious cases, obesity can contribute to angina pectoris and cardiac failure.

In addition to these medical conditions, there are other negative side effects to obesity. Adipose tissue around the chest and under the diaphragm interferes with respiration and creates a susceptibility to bronchitis. Breathing difficulty leads to retention of CO_2 (carbon dioxide) and subsequent sleepiness. Skin problems occur because of the excess deposits of fat underneath the skin, which is predisposed to infections. The folds and curves of the skin are especially susceptible to infection, particularly the area under women's breasts.

A Physiological Model of Obesity

Some researchers have theorized that fat cells control a "set point" weight in each person. When the fat cells become smaller, they send a message to the brain to ingest more food. Because an obese individual has more and larger fat cells, the obese person has an overwhelming urge to eat. This is why we often hear people who have been on diets talk about gaining back more weight than they first lost. The signal to eat becomes too powerful and the result is rebound overeating. The set point is raised and it now becomes more difficult to even maintain the previous weight.

Metabolic changes actually help maintain obesity and make the person more susceptible to weight gain after dieting. Once an obese person who has lost weight begins to eat again, the body produces and stores excess fat in its fat cells and liver, as if it is preparing itself for the possibility of another diet.

In 1995 researchers at Johns Hopkins Bayview Medical Center discovered a human gene mutation that predisposes an individual to obesity and accelerates the onset of Type II diabetes mellitus. The gene was found in the Pima Indians of Arizona, who have a very high incidence of both obesity and diabetes. The researchers have discovered this gene in 12 percent of white Americans and 25 percent of black Americans. Subsequent research in Finland, Sweden, and France supported this finding and concluded that the mutation may result in a lower metabolic rate, which leads to an accumulation of fat tissue in the abdominal region. This excess fat tissue has an influence in the development of insulin resistance, increased blood pressure, and diabetes. The researchers warn that carrying this gene doesn't guarantee that the person will be obese. Diet and exercise are still factors for this condition.

Psychological Model of Obesity

Obesity is one of the most challenging health conditions to treat. Our society values rich foods and dining out. Eating provides an opportunity to spend time with family and friends, sometimes the only time we can manage to spend with them because of our busy lifestyles and demanding jobs.

But eating can also be a solitary event, often associated with watching television. In terms of the psychological perspective of obesity, some people assume overeating happens as a result of external stimuli such as smell, taste, sight of food—even if the person is not hungry. Obese people are more likely to eat when involved in food-related activities. For example, watching television has been connected with the onset of obesity. The more television one watches, the greater one's degree of obesity. Of course, watching television also means decreased physical activity and a lower metabolic rate, which ultimately means that there is a decrease in the body's ability to burn fat.

Other psychological aspects of obesity have nothing to do with television. Typically, obese people have experienced some form of psychological trauma before or since they became obese. I will talk later about this trauma, but first I would like to address the negative implications of being obese. Unfortunately, obese people are discriminated against in employment opportunities, college entry, fashion, advertising, and even in relationships with family and friends. The social rejection of obese people contributes to a form of isolation in which "comfort foods" replace human contact. Couple this discrimination with being African-American, and we can see what almost 50 percent of African-American women live with day to day. These negative views about obesity, and therefore about oneself, create low self-esteem, self-deprecating attitudes that spiral into vicious cycles of depression, negative behavior, and more overeating. Without addressing the psychological component of obesity, no diet plan will ever be effective. Psychotherapy and homeopathy are two paths to achieving a healthy psychological outlook on obesity.

The following case is an example of the trauma that an obese person may experience. You will see how situations in her childhood created the need to be protected, to surround and insulate herself with a shield that took the form of excess weight. These same circumstances also helped develop her low self-esteem, which only worked to further increase her weight. Finally, you will hear about a most important and common aspect of this condition: the fear of getting well.

TWO CASES

Juanita is a very attractive, personable woman with a good sense of humor. The problem she had when she came to see me was with her weight. "I want to free myself of obesity," she told me on her first visit. "I weigh three hundred pounds and I'm only five feet tall. I'm ashamed of my body—that affects my sex life. I don't want to take my clothes off in front of other people. And all of the lights have to be off."

When I asked her more questions about her life, she began to open up about her deep-seated insecurities. "I have never liked myself," she admitted. "I have always seen myself as unattractive, even as a child. I want to be healthy now. I'm losing the fear of being healthy."

Juanita continued by telling me that her mother died when she was a teenager. Because she was the oldest of her siblings and the only girl, the family looked to her for guidance, and indirectly demanded that she be responsible at an early age. She felt burdened and resentful. She felt pressured and taken advantage of by her father. This resentment was particularly strong because he had not treated her mother well when she was alive. He often cheated on his wife and his steady stream of girlfriends provided Juanita's mother with a great cross to bear. "I felt my mother's pain all of the time." The humiliation and embarrassment from her father's actions were too much for her mother to handle.

But there were other sources of grief for Juanita. She was the only black child in her class, from kindergarten to sixth grade. "I was called nigger on a regular basis," she said. "It was horrible and frightening. I felt awkward. I felt ugly and different. I liked my inner self then, but not my physical self. I used to help everyone and be nice to everyone so that I could balance all of the negative feelings. I thought if I didn't give to others I would be useless, worthless, and ugly. I didn't think I'd be loved if I didn't give."

She told me all of this, and yet I felt she had not told me everything. Something was missing.

"Tell me more about your childhood, please," I said.

She began by telling me that at an early age she had been sexually abused. While the memories of that event were fragmented, she remembered that she began to put on additional weight when she was sexually abused for the second time by the same man. She remembered feeling it was her fault because she was well developed at a young age and she thought she had done something to attract the man. Part of this self-reproach came from the fact that she began masturbating as a child, and she thought it meant something was wrong with her. Looking back, she thought her masturbating two or three times a week was excessive at that age. Her sex drive and her masturbation made her too scared to tell her parents about the sexual abuse. She thought her parents would blame her for the situation. She was also afraid that her father would kill the man, because he was a trusted friend of the family.

After allowing her to weep for some time, I asked her what situation or circumstances frightened her as an adult. She lifted her head and said, "I fear being a normal weight." Fortunately, I had heard this same response many times before. The issue didn't revolve around weight. It revolved around the fear of being healthy again. The first time I encountered this type of response was during my first year of practice in Seattle. A young woman who had crippling arthritis told me she feared being well. She wondered what it would be like to date again, and to dance again—her favorite activity. But she was afraid of the possibility of failure, and her disability was a way of avoiding the situation. (Fear of healing is discussed elsewhere in this book.)

Juanita continued by explaining to me that when she lost weight in the past her family seemed jealous. They were unkind. They teased her and gave her little encouragement. She remembered crying constantly whenever this happened. Her family never recognized how challenging it was for her to exercise and eat differently. She had no support for her efforts. She not only regained her weight but added another twenty-five pounds.

"When I am overeating, I think I'm taking care of myself—food is love. I think to myself, 'What will I have in place of food?' I would have to stand up on my own two feet, I guess." Juanita seemed to be deeply disturbed by her circumstances, yet she seemed to have a grasp of the role of food in her life. "I am holding on to food like a baby to a pacifier. Doctors, especially men, do not understand the deeper issues of obesity. I am fat. I'm out of control and lack will power. It creates more shame. It is just a symptom of what is wrong, and they do not sit down and talk to you about it."

As with any patient, I prescribed the homeopathic remedy medor-rhinum in a 200 c potency, mainly because of her nature—extremes in personality, mood swings and early masturbation. I gave her a diet diary

and arranged for her to come back in three weeks. Medorrhinum reduces the need for extremes in one's behavior—in this case, overeating—and brings balance to the emotional and mental systems.

Like Juanita, Mary, a Caucasian American woman, came to me because of her weight. She too felt she was ugly and unacceptable, but for
different reasons. "I have tremendous stress and I haven't taken the
best care of myself," she said. "I've always been depressed. I'm forty
pounds overweight and I feel ashamed and burdened. I come from a
family that is addicted to alcohol. Food is a tool to comfort me. I don't
feel good about myself and I am in a cycle of not caring about myself.
My concentration is poor and I feel fuzzy-headed and spacey a lot of
times. I just don't like myself and there is nothing I can do to make me
feel good about myself. My weight makes it worse. I got divorced and
lost everything: that's part of my stress. I'm raising my children on my
own. My husband gives me nothing."

As I spent time with Mary, I realized her divorce was but the end
of a series of events that had chipped away at her self-esteem and security. When Mary was very young, her father committed suicide after he
and her mother separated. He was only twenty-eight years old. Her
mother remarried but her stepfather was "emotionally incapable" of
raising her. Her mother was alcoholic, and physically and verbally
abused her. "I was always the target of her rage and aggression," Mary
said. "I remember the pain, misery, and fear of my childhood. I was
disconnected from her. She treated me as if I was nobody." Mary began
to sob as she said, "She looked at me as defective. She was always trying
to remedy me. I was always being carted off to a psychologist or hospital
to get fixed."

Once when Mary's parents were out of town, she had a party. When
her mother discovered what she had done, she committed Mary to a
state mental hospital. The hospital was overcrowded and the therapist
suggested that the whole family needed therapy. But Mary's mother
would not hear of it and did not come back to the hospital. Mary remained there for three weeks. Her mother told her and the therapist
that Mary had inherited bad genes from her father. As a result, Mary
said, she was never sure of herself and always frightened. "I was brought
up to think I was different, but not in a positive way. Now I hide in
order to get by. I am cautious and untrusting, because I don't think
people like me. I went all through school and never said a word. I was

in the back row always thinking, 'Don't call on me.' I didn't want to be looked at or seen. I was fat, ugly, and stupid."

Mary's nature led her to believe that people did not like her and that she was essentially a bad person. Her complete lack of self-worth and -esteem in combination with her poor concentration and complaints of feeling spacey and anxious led me to prescribe the remedy Lac caninum in a 200 c potency.

The remedies prescribed for these women are not what I want to emphasize, however. Rather, I want to emphasize the psychology and need for something that introduces the concepts of self-love, not self-hate. The first step on the path to self-love is to recognize the problem and to be willing to seek assistance. The next step is uncovering the trauma in your life (trauma which does not have to be as severe as Mary's or Juanita's) in a structured, supportive setting, such as psychotherapy and homeopathy.

After explaining the diet diary to my overweight patients, I tell them three things:

1. The key to any healing is self-love, which begins with wanting what is best for ourselves. We have to want to love ourselves and heal ourselves, *for ourselves,* not for anyone else. Obesity is not different. We have to decide and want to lose weight for ourselves, not anyone else.

2. We have to commit ourselves for long-term healing and continued self-love, through the process of weight reduction. This means being patient with yourself and the process. Regardless of our weight, we must maintain a love for the self. Loving all parts of the self is the foundation for changing a negative self-image. Hating any part of the self will reinforce the negative image and establish excess weight even more firmly. Hating anything (or anyone) attaches that thing to you; it controls you.

3. There must be long-term (ultimately, a lifetime) commitment to changing behavior and relationships toward food. For example, we should eat when we are hungry. We should not eat if we are not hungry. Stop eating when full. As I said in Chapter 4, "Nutrition and Your Blood Type,"

there must be a change in circumstances under which food is eaten. Do not eat standing up or on the run. Do not watch television while eating because your attention will be divided and you will not feel as nourished. Do not eat when you are emotionally upset. Chew slowly and enjoy your food. Changing your relationship to food may also mean changing relationships. Choose to have some relationships with people who do not have food issues and who encourage you and support your goals and aspirations about your ideal body weight.

On her return visit, Juanita said to me, "I can see my eating is out of control. It was painful to write down how much I eat." Juanita's diet diary listed foods high in white flour, rice, sugar, saturated fats in the form of fried foods, potato chips, ice cream, pork, eggs, and soda. She ate minimal amounts of vegetables and fruits.

Juanita said she was aware of feeling calmer emotionally, having more mental clarity and sleeping better. We explored the reasons for her overeating and discovered that, aside from eating when she was premenstrual, the pressure of her job also made her overeat. Almost a year ago, her boss had added more responsibility and demands on her without additional compensation or job status. She could feel the racism as promotions sprang up around her. It brought back the pain of being called "nigger."

Mary recognized her coffee (with cream and sugar) addiction by the time she returned for a second visit. While she was mindful of eating vegetables, her diet diary reflected an excess of sodas, chips, and chocolate, and an inadequate amount of water. And equally as important, she noticed she only moved her bowels every other day. She said she was definitely feeling better psychologically.

During their return visits, I instructed both women on the foods and food preparation for the detox diet. Most importantly, I told each of them this was a cleansing diet, not necessarily a diet to lose weight. It was okay if they did not follow it perfectly. I made it clear that they could not fail on this diet because there were no demands. If they decided to drink sodas after ten days on the diet, that was fine with me. If they wanted to eat pork chops for one of the ten days, that was fine with me too. Whatever they did was fine with me. And if they did not do anything, that was fine with me too. I made it clear that, like anything else, what they put into the detox diet is what they get out. I also suggested that, if they had a real craving to eat a particular food, they should buy that food but eat it slowly. I suggested they avoid getting on a scale for several months.

Eight weeks passed. When Juanita returned, she felt more at peace with herself. She said she had been remarkably calm at work. "I look stronger, calmer, and more focused, and I feel that way." She had not exercised as much as she would have liked, but she was doing well with her diet, substituting more natural foods for those high in fat and salt and those with simple carbohydrates.

By Mary's third visit, approximately two and a half months later, she told me she felt awful for the first ten days after seeing me the first time (which can sometimes happen after a homeopathic remedy is given). "Everything was worse, but then I started feeling my old strength coming back. I feel good. I feel a definite easing of all the emotional issues. I have worked through things at my job that were burdening me about my coworkers not liking me. I do not feel as if I am in a secondary position anymore. I believe I can do something for myself. I am worthy."

Without these changes in mood and attitude, it is difficult to begin the process of weight loss. If you are depressed, angry, or anxious on a regular basis, you may use food to provide comfort and ease your tension. Once this pattern begins, fat cells enlarge and insulin sensitivity decreases. The more fat you have in your body, the higher the fasting insulin levels and the more likely you are to impair your blood sugar level tolerance by creating rebound hypoglycemia (a condition in which the blood sugar level is too low) and increased hunger. This insulin insensitivity affects food intake and weight regulation. And so the cycle of overeating begins.

GENERAL DIETARY SUGGESTIONS

Diets that promise you will lose thirty pounds in thirty days are neither healthy nor successful. Starvation or semistarvation and fad diets have been associated with medical risks. Starvation diets disrupt glucose tolerance and greatly reduce glucose levels in the body. Uric acid levels increase in the blood, while urinary output of uric acid decreases. Prolonged fasting also results in a loss of electrolytes—potassium, sodium, calcium, and magnesium. If you are diabetic or have any blood sugar imbalance, you should not fast. Besides these medical risks, you also will gain the weight back and add more weight to your frame. There is no diet that will work over the long term without reduced intake of energy (calories/food) and increased expenditure of energy (exercise). Most people will begin to lose weight if they decrease their caloric intake below 1500 calories per day and do aerobic exercise for twenty minutes, three or four times per week.

Behavior modification and psychological support are essential if you are obese or overweight. For that reason, the diet diary is an important tool to achieving reduced weight. Recording the foods you eat in a diet diary is necessary, albeit sometimes also painful, so that you can begin to see what, when, why and how much you are eating.

The detoxification diet is essential as a next step in changing your weight. It is designed to allow patients to increase their elimination by increasing the ingestion of fiber. Weight consists of fat and fat-free tissue, like minerals, electrolytes, glycogen, muscle, bone. It is also made up of waste and water content. By eliminating more waste and water from the body, you are reducing the inches and pounds.

Eating the foods on the detoxification diet also affords you the opportunity to see what it feels like to eat well, and to see what you feel like when you do not eat well. Very often the new feeling of wellness is enough to motivate people to change their lifestyle—to accommodate healthier habits. By "well" I mean that the diet encourages you to eat foods without chemicals—that means no preservatives, dyes, or pesticides—and to eat whole foods rather than refined foods that are low in nutrients.

Ideally, your diet should be high in dietary fiber (50 grams) and complex carbohydrates (60–70 percent of the total caloric content of your diet), with some protein (10–15 percent) and some fat (15–20 percent). Nutrition experts believe that a diet low in fiber and high in simple, refined carbohydrates is the major factor in obesity in the United States.

To reduce your set point, **refined carbohydrates (white flour) and saturated fats must be totally eliminated from your diet.** Fats have approximately 9 calories per gram, as compared with 4 calories per gram for proteins and carbohydrates. Reducing fat intake alone will result in significant weight loss. In a 1200-calorie-a-day diet, you should only be consuming about 180 calories from fat, which is approximately 20 grams a day. Concentrated sugars (including honey, fruit juices, and dried fruit) should be no more than 10 percent of your caloric intake.

Aside from helping eliminate excess waste and water from the body, the increased dietary fiber in your diet will affect your weight for several other reasons. First, fiber increases the amount of necessary chewing and therefore slows the eating process, allowing more time for digestion of food. Fiber also increases the excretion of fat in the feces. Third, as I discussed in Chapter 7, "Diabetes," fiber improves the body's glucose tolerance, which in turn affects how efficiently the body uses its energy. Finally, fiber stimulates the release of intestinal hormones, which make the individual feel more satisfied and sated. Because fiber plays such an important role in a proper diet, it may be necessary to add a fiber supplement, but no more than 5 grams, in divided doses per day.

In order to maintain a healthy diet, it is also important to eat meals at specific times. Snacking is deadly. Studies have shown that a healthy person who is dieting demonstrates the eating pattern of someone who is obese. When given foods to snack on, these average-weight dieters ate more food during the meal immediately after snacking than those average-weight people who were not dieting. Likewise, obese people were found to eat larger meals after snacking than if they had eaten nothing.

Snacking on sugary products is one of the most damaging habits on a successful diet. Insulin secretion is 70 percent greater after eating a candy bar, for example, than consuming the same number of calories from something nutritious, like a peanut-raisin snack. The candy bar, a simple carbohydrate, will cause immediate increases in blood sugar levels and insulin secretion in direct relation to its number of calories. This aggravates a person's obesity by creating a rapid descent in blood sugar level (hypoglycemia) and encouraging subsequent hunger.

It is still of primary importance to follow the diet appropriate for your blood type. Generally, women need approximately 2000 calories a day and men need about 2500 calories. Along with eight to ten glasses of water per day to flush the system and reduce hunger, you should aim for eating approximately 1200 calories per day if you hope to lose one to three pounds per week. By multiplying ideal body weight in kilograms (2.2 pounds per kilogram) by the following calories, you can assess your dietary caloric requirement, depending on your level of activity.

Sedentary: 30 calories
Light physical activity: 35 calories
Moderate physical activity: 40 calories
Heavy physical activity: 45 calories

In other words, an 80-kg (176-pound) man who exercises moderately needs 3200 calories per day in order to maintain his weight. (80 kgs × 40 calories = 3200 calories.)

One pound of fat represents about 3500 excess calories. To lose one pound a week, you have to have a negative calorie intake of 3500 per week, or 500 calories a day. A 1200- to 1500-calorie diet means you may enjoy 9–10 servings (½ cup equals a serving) of sauteed, steamed, or grilled vegetables, 4–6 servings of fruit (1 fruit, or 3-to-5 ounces per serving), 5–6 servings of bread (1 slice per serving), cereals (½ to ¾ cup) and starchy vegetables like corn (⅔ cup), sweet potatoes (¼ cup), white potatoes (1 small), butternut or acorn squash (½ cup), or parsnips (⅔ cup). One or two ½-cup servings of beans, 2 servings (1-ounce) of lean lamb, veal, chicken, turkey, or fish are excellent sources of protein. Oils such as sunflower, safflower, canola, grapeseed, and olive may be used for fats, along with butter. But you should use no more than 4 or 5 servings (1 teaspoon per serving) a week.

As I said earlier, if you want to lose weight, you must make a long-term commitment to this process. As I also said, no diet will work without reduced energy intake (eating) and increased energy output (exercising). While the commitment must be to *do* both, *the most important commitment is to yourself.*

EXERCISE

Exercise is a critical part of the weight loss program. While you may lose weight while dieting, you are more likely to lose fat-free tissue like electrolytes and muscular tissue than fat tissue if you do not also exercise regularly. For all blood types, the exercise does not have to be strenuous, but it does have to be a form of exercise that requires endurance three times a week for twenty to sixty minutes, at an intensity of 60 percent of your maximum heart rate. If you are blood type A, you will still find it necessary to do yoga or tai chi for the purpose of relaxing the mind, but you will need aerobic exercise for weight loss.

It is better to exercise moderately for a longer period of time than to expend a lot of energy for a short period of time. Start with a brisk walk for twenty to thirty minutes daily. Ultimately, your exercise should include any activity that uses large muscle groups, that can be maintained continuously, and that requires rhythmic, aerobic work, such as jogging, bicycling, rebounding, jumping rope, rowing, or stair climbing. In order to lose weight, you need to use these techniques while exercising twenty to forty minutes per day at least three times a week.*

HERBAL TREATMENTS AND NUTRITIONAL SUPPLEMENTS

Herbs and nutritional supplements help break down fat tissue in obese patients. Two herbs I use frequently for this purpose are *Ephedra sinica* and *Camellia sinensis.*

Ephedra has been used in China since approximately 2800 B.C. It is used primarily for asthma, bronchitis and hypotension (low blood pressure). In the early 1900s ephedra found its way into pharmaceutical companies when people realized that one of its chemical constituents, ephedrine, had druglike effects. Specifically, ephedra acts like epinephrine, a hormone that is secreted by the adrenal glands primarily in response to low blood sugar. It stimulates the sympathetic nervous system, and therefore stimulates the contraction of the blood vessels, increases blood pressure and flow, stimulates the heart, and relaxes smooth muscles of the bronchi. Ephedrine promotes weight loss by increasing the metabolic rate of the adipose (fat) tissue and diminishing appetite. Individuals with low metabolic rates have the greatest results from ephedrine. Ephedrine is also known to work more effectively in combination with caffeine and theophylline (also known as methylxanthines), and though I am not promoting the consumption of coffee, caffeine in other

---

*Aerobic exercise changes the set point I spoke of earlier and burns calories.

forms helps with the promotion of weight loss. A final word of caution about ephedra: you should be careful when taking this herb because it may cause hypertension, anxiety, and insomnia. I recommend 1 gram per day in divided doses.

Camellia sinensis, or green tea, contains caffeine and is the herb I use in combination with ephedra for the purpose of weight loss. The caffeine enhances the increased metabolic rate and fat cell and fat cell breakdown due to ephedra. When used alone, however, green tea has no significant effect on weight loss. It is, remember, extremely rich in flavonoids, which have very potent antioxidant and antiallergy properties. I recommend one cup of green tea per day.

Fat cells contain two different receptors: one for hormones that inhibit fat decomposition and one for those that stimulate decomposition. Therefore, blocking the cells that inhibit fat disintegration promotes the removal of fat from the cells. These particular receptors are more common in the fat cells of the breasts, buttocks and thighs. Since these sites are particularly resistant to weight loss, it is particularly useful to block the receptor sites in these areas.

Corynanthe yohimbe (yohimbine), another herb I use to treat obesity, blocks these fat cell receptors, while enhancing fat cell splitting and decomposition and decreasing appetite. With hypertensive patients, I start with very low doses of the liquid form of the herb because, like ephedra, it may cause anxiety and insomnia. I also warn patients not to have fermented foods like red wine and beer, or foods with high contents of tyramine, like cabbage, cheese, and potatoes, when they are taking yohimbine. Start with 1 mg, three times a day. Increase the dosage by 1 mg in three-week intervals. If there are toxic effects, decrease the amount and begin again at lower doses. Do not exceed 18 mg per day.

A final note about obesity. In most overweight or obese patients, the liver does not function effectively. The liver aids in the breakdown and metabolism of fat. To improve this function, I prescribe the herb *Taraxacum* or dandelion root. Dandelion decreases liver congestion by aiding in the removal of fat from the liver and in helping to decrease the accumulation of fat. It increases both production of bile by the liver and the flow of bile to the gall bladder. Also, stimulation of the gall bladder by dandelion causes the gall bladder to contract and release the bile into the intestine, where it can emulsify fat. I generally prescribe 4 grams of the dried powder or 500–1000 mg of solid extract.

Taking responsibility for and making a commitment to yourself is the foundation of empowerment, taking charge, and creating success in your life. It starts with you. Once that is accomplished, you are more capable of creating success in your world.

I believe we can do anything we truly want and commit to do. But we often want a reward, we want to know what is in it for us. The rewards for losing weight are obvious—a higher quality of life. You will feel better because you will be less restricted in movement and activity and less prone to the complications of obesity. Greater confidence and self-esteem are other obvious rewards. You will no longer be self-conscious with every step you take or be afraid to enter into a new place or group for fear of ridicule or embarrassment. Your life will be richer with the thoughts of knowing what you have accomplished and the discipline you have gained as a result.

Consider Mr. William J. Cobb, written about in the July 30, 1963, *Time* magazine. Mr. Cobb weighed 802 lbs and could eat fifteen chickens in one sitting. After patience and perseverance, on a 1000-calorie-a-day diet for 83 weeks, he lost 570 lbs! If Mr. Cobb can do it, so can you.

9

ARTHRITIS

TWO CASES

"I have numbness and pain when I lie down. Besides the arthritis, I have diabetes and hypertension. I've had two back surgeries. My thumbs ache and are stiff all the time. It's worse in the right hand. I'm afraid I'll just freeze up. For a while I thought I had MS [multiple sclerosis] or something."

This woman, whom I will call Helen, explained to me that her boyfriend had died six years previously from autoimmune deficiency syndrome (AIDS). He contracted the human immunodeficiency virus (HIV) from a blood transfusion he received for complications from an automobile accident. For nearly ten years she cared for his broken bones and internal injuries and then for his virus. She would often have to nurse him day and night. On some weeks she would have to give him nightly injections to alleviate the pain. Sometimes she would just have to sit with him because he asked her to. Sleep for her was often nonexistent or sporadic at best.

During those years Helen raised two children, attended to all of their needs, and for the most part ignored her own. She constantly worried about her finances and her boyfriend's illness. A very faithful and religious woman, she asked God and God alone for help. Only God would give her boyfriend relief and quiet him down. Then she could get some rest.

She realized now that she was in need of help. But then she didn't think about it; she didn't ask for help and no one offered. "Now," she said, "my body is just plain worn out."

Despite the problems in their lives, her relationship was good. She felt bonded to him. When he was diagnosed with HIV, however, the relationship suffered considerable amounts of strain. But particularly it suffered because she was afraid to have sexual relations with him. He became angry, often cursing and hollering at her, and occasionally throwing things around the room. But never once did he hit her.

"I wanted it to be over, but I didn't want to let him go," she admitted.

Finally she had to let him go. When that day came, she felt physical pain, "like I was cut in half with a knife." Ultimately, the pain and grief subsided. Then began the process of forgiveness of herself for judging his behavior as being selfish and unloving. She had a lot of bitterness, not just about their relationship the last three years of his life, but also because of the things that had happened throughout the relationship. She also felt angry about his death and watched violent movies to release the anger.

Helen told me she felt as she did when she was a child: shy, quiet, and reluctant to talk to people because she didn't think she could hold a conversation. Besides, she said, she was a private person, keeping things to herself except for maybe occasionally confiding in her sister. "I don't trust others enough to tell them anything. I don't trust them to keep things in confidence or to understand."

"What was your childhood like?" I asked. She told me she was not allowed to have much interaction with other kids. She was a private person, with just one or two friends. She didn't like crowds and didn't like holding a conversation with people she didn't know.

Her father wasn't home much and when he was home he simply gave the children orders. She was beaten so badly by her father that her mother took him to court. But it left a permanent scar on Helen because she could no longer trust men, much less expect anything from them. It was not until after becoming a Christian and learning how to forgive that was she able to have a good relationship.

When she came to see me, Helen's arthritis was her greatest concern. The balls of her thumbs ached. Lifting and turning things were difficult. Whatever side she would lie on at night would ache and become numb after a few hours, causing her to toss and turn in bed. The pain down her leg would feel better if she were lying on her left side. Yet any movement, such as walking or even sitting, made this pain worse.

Helen was always thirsty and suffered from constipation. Her diet was comprised of chicken, colas, chips, apple pie, brownies, sausage and egg sandwiches from a fast food chain, and an occasional vegetable.

While no longer depressed about her boyfriend or her life, Helen was often irritable, stubborn, and opinionated. I believe that her arthritis, worry about survival and finances, moods, along with her need to be a private person, called for the remedy *Bryonia alba*. I gave her a low potency of this medication to take daily and sent her home with a diet diary to record her food for five days.

Helen's diet diary reflected that she did eat exactly what she said— very low-fiber foods, few vegetables, excess sweets and colas, and fast food. The way she responded to the mental and emotional stress of her life and her nutritional habits made it clear to me how she became susceptible to disease, in this case arthritis.

Another patient of mine, Sheila, was diagnosed with systematic lupus erythematosus and polyarthritis (arthritis in multiple joints) at a very low point in her life. She had quit school, was without work and was receiving public assistance. She felt like she was at a "dead end." The first signs of her condition were painful, stiff, and swollen fingers and knees. (And though she was currently on prednisone and Plaquenil, she still had pain and stiffness.) Although they eventually became husband and wife, the man with whom she lived at the time of the onset of her condition, was not willing to marry or be as supportive as she needed for him to be. She felt dependent and needy because of her pain and disability.

Being dependent and needy was not foreign to Sheila. "I felt like I was nothing unless I accomplished something," she said. "I never felt like I was important to my parents. I would tiptoe around my parents for fear of doing something wrong. I was squelched by my father's personality. I had to do what he thought was best, because he was very concerned about public appearances and impressing others. My mother was cold, distant, and not at all affectionate. She did not spend much time with me. I always had to be and look a certain way. I couldn't be who I wanted to be; I had to be what they always wanted and always be in control of myself." Sheila's father was verbally abusive and she was still concerned that people would retaliate verbally and humiliate her if she confronted them or stood up for herself.

"I felt I was nothing. I was just a victim. I still worry about what to say, how to dress, or whether I have made the right decision. I have always had an identity problem. I am always looking for who I am."

Sheila's husband is similar to her father in that he too is sometimes verbally abusive. "He drinks a lot, especially on vacation. When he drinks he wants to argue. Mostly he screams and hollers." While he has never hit her, these experiences are frightening for her. She told me she suppresses her feelings, especially her anger about her father, her husband, and her condition. But she can be short-tempered and she will throw things and curse a lot if provoked. She gets particularly angry when people take advantage of her and others.

Another source of pain for her was being childless. While in college, Sheila had an abortion because the man she was with decided he did not want her or the baby. As she cried, she told me of a second abortion she had while married to her husband. That time she aborted because of a health risk due to all of the drugs she was taking at the time. "I am a family-oriented person and I couldn't imagine life without children. When I see other people with children I feel left out."

Insomnia was another concern. It was very hard for Sheila to get to sleep. At times, sleep did not come until three or four in the morning. Once she was asleep, she had very vivid dreams of being chased by criminals with guns. Other dreams were of being threatened by storms and abandoned and ignored by others.

I prescribed for Sheila the remedy staphysagria, for her suppressed anger, feelings of abandonment, false sense of being "nothing," fears of conflict, inability to stand up for herself, insomnia, and grief. The experiences that created Sheila's nature led to the susceptibility to lupus and, thus, the arthritis.

What Is Arthritis?

"Arthur," as it is referred to by the black elderly, is the diagnosis for one out of every seven people in America. In simple terms, arthritis is an inflammation of the joints. It usually involves a synovial joint, a capsule consisting of synovial fluid and connective tissue that attaches one bone to another so that movement can occur. Cartilage is located at the ends of the bones and a membrane secretes fluid inside the joint. All of this is encased by a joint capsule, which keeps the joint in place. In an arthritic joint, the processes of wear and tear and regeneration are out of balance. There may not be enough synovial fluid, causing stiffness, or there may be too much, causing swelling. If the cartilage is worn, the bone rubs on bone, causing more pain. Arthritis can be a hereditary condition or the result of an injury or overuse. Infection and autoimmune disease may also cause arthritis.

Three of the more common types of and treatments for arthritis will be discussed in this chapter.

OSTEOARTHRITIS

Osteoarthritis, the most common form of arthritis, is caused mainly by progressive degeneration of the cartilage from wear and tear on the joint, and because of the inability of the body to regenerate the cartilage at the same pace. Over 40 million Americans have osteoarthritis, including 80 percent of persons over fifty. For those under the age of forty-five, osteoarthritis is more common among men.

Aspirin and nonsteroidal inflammatory drugs, like Advil or Motrin, impair the regeneration process because they impede growth of cartilage. The joints of the hips, knees, fingers, and spine are especially affected. Some of the telltale signs of this condition are stiffness, limited range of motion, cracking of the joints, and pain of motion.

Joint degeneration can also be caused by some inherited physical abnormality in the joint structure, inflammatory diseases like rheumatoid arthritis or gout, and trauma—from obesity or fractures. The conditions damage the cartilage, and the result is osteoarthritis.

RHEUMATOID ARTHRITIS

RA affects 3 percent of the population, mainly those between the ages of twenty and forty. Female RA patients outnumber male patients three to one. We know that RA is an autoimmune reaction (the immune system turns against the body and antibodies are produced against parts of the joint tissue) that attacks joints as well as skin and muscles. But it is a complicated disease. Experts do not know the exact cause of the autoimmune response, although they have many reasons: genetics, abnormal bowel walls (excess permeability, so that proteins leak into the blood), lifestyle and nutritional factors, microorganisms, and food allergies.

Some of the signs of RA include severe joint pain, with inflammation beginning in the small joints on hands, feet, and ankles (and often symmetrical on the body). The inflammation eventually progresses to all joints and leads to joint stiffness, fatigue, low-grade fever, weakness. X-ray findings will reveal erosion of the cartilage and narrowing of the joint space. The joints will usually be warm and tender. The skin over the joint will have a red-purplish color. Blood tests can confirm the presence of antibodies associated with the disease.

GOUT

Gout is caused by increased amounts of uric acid in the blood, a by-product of the metabolism of purines (see Glossary) made by the body and found in foods. The crystals of sodium urate form in the joints, tendon, kidneys and other tissues and cause severe pain and inflammation. The disease affects approximately one million Americans—mostly men. Women develop gout later in life because their uric acid levels rise when estrogen levels drop during menopause.

Called the "rich man's disease" because it is associated with men who have diets high in red meat and wine, gout often attacks in the middle of the night, after an evening of purine-rich foods like meats, or substances like alcohol that prevent the kidney from excreting uric acid. Gout does not happen overnight, however, and may take years to build up crystals for an attack. Usually the first attack is in one joint—the big toe. And because gout can be controlled by diet, the incidence of chronic gout in this country is relatively low.

People with gout are typically obese, prone to diabetes and hypertension, and at a high risk for heart disease. Low-dose aspirin therapy and some diuretic high blood pressure medications can also cause secondary gout.

HERBAL TREATMENTS
AND NUTRITIONAL SUPPLEMENTS

Herbal treatments don't just ease the pain—they help with the body's regeneration process. Herbs, in other words, help the body heal itself. Many herbs possess anti-inflammatory actions while others enhance the function and secretion of the body's own cortisone.

The more effective herbs for osteoarthritis, rheumatoid arthritis, and gout are discussed below.

HERBS FOR OSTEOARTHRITIS

The higher incidence of OA in women suggests that estrogen may play a role in this condition. Some herbs are used to treat OA because they have an ability to bind estrogen receptors in women. *Glycyrrhiza glabra,* or licorice root, inhibits estrogen activity if levels are too high and encourages activity if levels are too low. For some patients, I use 15 drops of this tincture three times a day. Or I give patients dry root powder to use 2 grams a day. (Consult a physician before using any more than this amount, especially if you have a history of hypertension, renal failure, or if you are on cardiac glycosides.) *Medicago sativa* is another herb I use that binds estrogen receptors.

I use other herbs to decrease inflammation. *Curcuma longa* (curcumin), or turmeric, is a most effective anti-inflammatory herb. Curcumin not only increases the secretion of our own cortisol (the body's answer to cortisone) but also sensitizes receptors for adrenal hormones, which makes these hormones more effective as an anti-inflammatory agent. Curcumin also stabilizes white cell membranes so they do not release inflammatory chemicals as easily, and stops the production of leukotriene (a substance produced by white blood cells that causes inflammation). I typically use curcumin in capsule form and prescribe 400 mg, three times a day.

Harpagphytum procumbens, or the devil's claw, possesses an anti-inflammatory and pain-killing effect. I use 1 to 2 grams, three times a day, on OA patients. *Zingiber officinale,* or ginger, also acts as an anti-inflammatory. I sometimes prescribe ginger as a tea. I tell the patient to grate 1 teaspoon of fresh ginger into a cup of hot water and drink 2 cups a day. Ginger tea may also be used as a hot compress to ease the pain and swelling of joints.

Crataegus oxyacantha, or hawthorn berries—besides being an excellent tonic for the heart—can enhance the integrity and stability of the collagen matrix, the main substance found in cartilage. The flavonoid molecules in the berries are what give the berries their red-blue color and provide anti-inflammatory activity. I prescribe 15 drops, two times per day.

Boswellia serrata is a gum resin found in certain trees in India. In addition to being an anti-inflammatory herb, it also increases blood supply to the joints, thus promoting healing. The dosage is 400 mg, three times a day.

There are several nutritional supplements I have my patients take as well.

- The most important supplement is **glucosamine sulphate**, a substance found inside the joints that aids in the formation of cartilage. The body produces glucosamine sulphate, but as we age we begin to produce smaller amounts. Glucosamine sulphate diffuses slowly from the blood into the bones. The typical dosage is 500 mg, three times a day.

- **Niacinamide** (B3) is another very important supplement. High doses have had good clinical results with patients suffering from OA, but there can be significant side effects dealing with the liver. B3 is necessary to prevent pellagra (dermatitis, diarrhea, psychological disturbances). I recommend 500 mg, two or three times a day, but I always closely monitor the liver enzymes to avoid harmful side effects.

- **Vitamin E** at 600 to 800 mg per day helps inhibit specific enzymes that break down the proteins of cartilage. It also increases the body's deposit of proteoglycans, one of the valuable components of cartilage. Vitamin E is also one of our most effective antioxidants (a substance that prevents oxidation of cell membranes and therefore prevents damage to the cell), which in turn helps prevent damage to our cartilage.

- **Vitamin C** is necessary for collagen synthesis and connective tissue repair. Vitamins C and E work better together than separately. The usual dosage is 1000–3000 mg per day, in divided doses.

- **Methionine** is a sulfur-containing amino acid which is critical in cartilage structures. In clinical trials, it also has proven to be more effective than ibuprofen in the treatment of OA, especially in relieving pain and increasing activity in the hip or knee areas.

Generally speaking, OA patients should be taking a high-quality multiple vitamin on a daily basis. That multivitamin should include at least 6 mg of **boron**, a mineral necessary for the formation and maintenance of cartilage. It should also have adequate amounts of **vitamin A, pyridoxine** (B6), as well as **zinc** and **copper**. If you do not take a multivitamin, go to a health food store and ask for their best brand. You are worth it!

RHEUMATOID ARTHRITIS

Ginger, curcumin, devil's claw, and licorice root I also use to treat RA. Chinese traditional medicine offers another herb called *Bupleurum falcatum,* the root of which is particularly useful for inflammatory conditions. The components of this root are like steroids, in that they increase the release of glucocorticoid hormones by the adrenal glands. Yet they do not cause the adrenal gland atrophy that is a common side effect of steroid drug use. Taking 2 to 4 grams of this herb per day is recommended.

Panax ginseng is a Korean herb that is referred to as an adoptogen, and agent that helps maintain homeostasis during periods of stress. Specifically, ginseng protects against mental and physical fatigue by influencing the adrenal glands. Ginseng helps to adjust metabolic systems of the body to create greater endurance and increased energy. As with the herb bupleurum, ginseng does not cause adrenal shrinkage. I prescribe 500 mg, two times a day.

Chinese skullcap or *Scutellaria baicalensis* has antiarthritic and anti-inflammatory powers similar in effect to indomethacin, a popular drug for the diagnosis of RA. The flavonoids in this herb inhibit the formation of leukotrienes and make it a potent antioxidant.

Hawthorn berries, or *Crataegus oxyacantha,* are a rich source of flavonoids that help stabilize the joint membranes and collagen, while promoting antioxidant and anti-inflammatory activity.

I also recommend to RA patients a host of nutritional supplements:

- ·⦿· Eicosapentaenoic acid (EPA) from fish oils—1 gram
- ·⦿· Vitamin E—400 IU, two times a day
- ·⦿· Methionine—500 mg, three times a day
- ·⦿· Niacinamide—500 mg, three times a day

- Quercetin—250 mg between meals, three times a day
- Vitamin C—1–3 gms per day in divided doses
- Selenium—200 mcg per day
- Zinc—45 mg per day
- Copper—1 mg per day
- Bromelain—250 mg (2000 mcu) between meals, three times a day
- Betaine HCL (hydrochloric acid)—5–10 grains with meals

Eicosapentaenoic acid, or omega-3 polyunsaturated fatty acid, reduces inflammation and relieves stiffness and pain. As with any form of natural healing, the benefits are not immediate. So be patient. After four to six months of taking 1 to 2 grams a day, you should notice significant improvement. This amount of oil is equivalent to approximately 4 ounces of cold-water fish (discussed in the General Dietary Suggestions on pp. 184–85) per day.

Quercetin, a flavonoid, helps to neutralize the inflammatory response. It inhibits the release of histamine from mast cells and basophils, thereby reducing the inflammatory activity in the body. Quercetin stabilizes the cell membranes and neutralizes free radicals (molecules that react with oxygen and cause oxidative damage to cells, proteins, and even DNA). It also inhibits many steps in the production of pro-inflammatory prostaglandins and leukotrienes.

Selenium is a trace mineral that reduces inflammation in patients who have low selenium levels. It stimulates the activity of the enzyme that neutralizes free radicals and improves the production of pro-inflammatory prostaglandins. The neutralizing of oxygen-free radicals is very important because those free radicals damage the synovial tissues (which surround the joints) and destroy the substance that lubricates the joints.

Zinc is also an antioxidant and, along with **copper**, is commonly in low levels in RA patients. Copper helps the body produce cartilage and collagen. Again, a good multivitamin/mineral supplement will have adequate amounts of both.

Bromelain is a wonderful combination of proteolytic enzymes found in the stem of a pineapple plant. I use it to provide relief for joint pain. I also use it for sinusitis and thrombophlebitis (blood clot in the leg). It inhibits pro-inflammatory prostaglandins, promotes the production of anti-inflammatory (series I) prostaglandins, and inhibits the increase in permeability of blood vessels that cause edema (swelling).

Low gastric acidity has been associated with RA. Proper digestion requires adequate amounts of **hydrochloric acid** in the stomach. Proteins especially need adequate amounts of hydrochloric acid to be digested. Impaired digestion can lead to allergic reactions throughout the body. Digestion also determines the maintenance of proper bowel flora, which is essential for immune system functioning and for optimal vitamin absorption.

GOUT

Diet, which will be discussed in General Dietary Suggestions (see below), is effective in reducing the incidence of gout. But herbal and nutritional supplements are usually necessary. I prescribe **eicosapentaenoic acid** (1–2 grams per day), **vitamin E** (400–800 IU per day), **vitamin C** (2000–4000 mg a day in divided doses), **folic acid** (10–40 mg per day), **bromelain** (125–250 mg, three times a day between meals, and **quercetin** (125–250 mg, three times a day between meals).

Devil's claw is the primary herb I prescribe for gout patients because it reduces serum cholesterol and uric acid levels. It also has a pain-killing effect. I prescribe 1–2 grams of this powder, three times a day, or 10 drops of the tincture, three times a day.

The only nutrient that has not been discussed is folic acid. Folic acid is useful because it inhibits the enzyme that produces uric acid. But high levels of folic acid can interfere with epilepsy drugs and can mask the signs of B12 deficiency.

Finally, a word of caution: high doses of niacin, above 50 mg per day, work against the body. Niacin decreases the excretion of harmful uric acids.

GENERAL DIETARY SUGGESTIONS

All of the dietary recommendations in Chapter 4, "Nutrition and Your Blood Type," should be implemented in your treatment plan to reduce problems from arthritis and to promote healing. You must avoid all simple, processed (refined), and concentrated carbohydrates. Place your emphasis on complex carbohydrates (whole foods) and high-fiber foods. Your diet must be low in red meat (if you are blood type O) and saturated fats. Plants from the Solanaceae family (see Glossary) should be eliminated—that includes tomatoes, white potatoes, eggplant, green peppers, and tobacco. Eliminating any food allergens is useful for any disease, but food allergies can especially aggravate RA. Common allergens include corn, wheat, and dairy products.

If you are supposed to eat animal protein, I recommend specific fish such as salmon, mackerel, halibut, herrings, and sardines. These fish have great amounts of eicosapentaenoic acid, which competes with arachidonic acid for prostaglandin production. If you are not eating enough fish or are a blood type A, you may try supplementing your diet with cod liver oil. You should also eat berries that are rich in flavonoids, such as blueberries, hawthorn berries, blackberries, and cherries. Those who have gout should consider eliminating alcohol and red meat completely, and drinking 6–8 eight-ounce glasses of water a day.

An interesting note in general, rheumatoid arthritis and gout are not found in societies that eat a more "primitive" diet of whole foods and few meats.

HOMEOPATHIC REMEDIES

By now you are aware that I treat people, not diseases. Any homeopathic remedy can be useful in the healing of arthritis. There are times, however, that it is essential to treat an acute situation—and even then we must consider the person's mood and temperament. Some homeopathic remedies for arthritis include:

- **Bryonia.** The joints are red, hot, and swollen and the knee joints are stiff and painful. The pain through the joints feels like a stitching or tearing pain and gets worse without motion. With all of the mucous membranes drying out, the patient will be thirsty. The patient also exhibits extreme irritability.
- **Caulophyllum** is useful for the pain and stiffness of the fingers or toes, especially if the fingers are the only joints affected. The joint pains are severe and erratic. Wrists may ache and hands may feel cutting pain when closed into a

fist. The pains can also change places every few minutes. Joint pains are worse before menses and better after the flow.

❧ **Causticum** is used for arthritis of the hands and fingers, especially if the pain is worse while bathing or in cold or dry weather. It is also useful for gout. The patient may experience a weakness in the ankles and unsteady walking. The knees may crack and feel stiff in the hollow. The temperament for this condition is one of extreme sympathy for others.

❧ **Colchicum** is the plant used for the medication colchicine, which is the drug of choice for gout. The homeopathic preparation of colchicum is also used for gout. The joints will become severely inflamed and get worse without motion. Merely touching the joint with anything may be too painful for the patient. Pains travel from the left to right side of the body, and patients can experience tearing pains in warm weather and in the evening. The smell of food can create nausea and one's thirst is almost always unquenchable. The mood of these patients is of someone who is anxious, irritable, sad, and fretful.

❧ **Gauiacum** is useful for gout and arthritic pains that feel better from cold applications and worse from heat and motion. The joint feels hot or even burning. Left wrist pain, or carpal tunnel syndrome, is also an indication for guaiacum. If you need this remedy, you may also be stubborn, sullen, fretful, and arrogant.

❧ *Kalmia latifolia* is a remedy used for people who have arthritis that moves downward on the body. The pain usually moves from hips to knees to the feet. The pains are sudden, severe and acute, worse at night and with motion. The limbs are often weak, numb, and cold. There is pain along the ulnar nerve of the forearm and in the index finger. People needing kalmia may be anxious and have a feeling that something bad will happen to them. They have little motivation and desire for work.

❧ **Ledum** is for people who have gouty pains that shoot all through the foot, limb, and joints, especially small joints.

The knee can be affected as well. Swelling of the foot and ankle is common. The joint can be swollen, hot, and pale. The pain begins in the lower limbs and ascends. There is a tremendous desire to put the foot in cold or ice water. All the pains are worse from being overheated in bed. The person may be angry, irritable, and discontented.

❧ **Pulsatilla** is known for wandering arthritis—arthritis that moves around the body. Drawing pains in the hips and thighs with restlessness is indicative of the need for this remedy. The pains are worse during first motion but are alleviated with more movement and with cold temperatures, and worse in warmer conditions. The knees may be swollen, as are the veins in the forearms, hands, and legs. The person may be emotional, weep easily, and crave sympathy. A mild disposition indicates pulsatilla.

❧ *Rhus toxicodendron* aids patients with hot, painful joints that swell in cold, damp weather but are relieved by hot baths. The pain increases with exertion. The person can be hurried and impatient, and either cheerful or irritable.

EXERCISE AND PHYSICAL MEDICINE

You may think that having arthritis means you don't have to exercise. Quite the contrary. Exercise is one of the most important therapies for arthritis. If you don't exercise, the pain becomes worse because the joints stiffen and muscles and ligaments around the joints weaken.

Daily nontraumatic exercise, such as isometrics (in which muscles are tensed against other muscles or against an immovable object so that they contract without shortening) and swimming, is extremely important. Strengthening and passive range-of-motion exercises (where you or someone else takes your joints through its range of motion) are also important for maintaining joint function. As the inflammation is reduced, active range-of-motion exercises (in which you use your own strength to move your joint through its range of motion) and isotonic exercises (in which you use light weights as you move the joint through its range of motion) will be appropriate.

Examples of range-of-motion exercises include looking directly down at the ground with your neck bent; bending your neck directly back; turning your head to left and right; putting your left ear to your left shoulder and then your right ear to your right shoulder; making a tight fist, then opening your hand after the count to 10 and extending your fingers, making them as wide apart as you can; bending your elbows; raising your arms above your head, stretching gently and lowering them; and raising and lowering your hands at your wrists. These exercises should be done in repetitions of 10, one or two times a day. If you don't know any exercises to do, ask you physician or physical therapist.

The benefits of exercise are obvious. Exercise strengthens the muscles around the joints, thereby providing greater support for the joint. Weight control through regular exercise alleviates stress to the joints. Without regular exercise, the nutrients and blood flow to the joints are limited, as is the healing for the joints. As was discussed in Chapter 4, "Nutrition and Your Blood Type," the best preventive care for osteoporosis, a condition related to arthritis, is to exercise. Stressing the bone through exercise helps keep it dense and strong. Putting your joints through full range-of-motion exercises keeps the joints mobile. Remember not to overdo it, to breathe while exercising, and to rest when you need to.

There are physical medicine therapies I tell some arthritic patients to use. Generally, for acute flareups, I recommend they apply cold packs or ice packs to the joints. But to get nutrients and blood flowing to the joint for healing and repair, moist heat is more effective than dry heat. Hot baths, hot moist packs, and paraffin (wax as used by manicurists or reflexologists) baths are particularly effective to increase circulation and promote healing. Cayenne powder, which stimulates circulation, may be used as part of the hot, moist pack, by putting a cloth in a solution of hot water and powder. Massage, whether on the whole body or only on the joints, will increase circulation. Warm castor oil used during massages will increase body mobility. And whole body massages also relieve pain by affecting the mind and nervous system.

So what happened to the patients I introduced at the beginning of this chapter? It has been almost two years since I first saw Sheila. During that time she has consistently improved. Within the fist month she told me, "I already feel better emotionally because I am taking control of my health now. Before, I was at the mercy of conventional doctors and they would just laugh at me. They did not take me seriously. I don't want to rely solely on prescription drugs." She was still having a hard time falling asleep, but the time was reduced to one hour of restlessness rather than four or five.

Since becoming a patient in my office, she has not had an acute attack of lupus. A year after her first visit, she told me, "Usually I have a flareup at least once or twice a year. I am doing really well. The pain and stiffness are gone. I've eliminated the Plaquenil and cut down considerably on the prednisone—from 10 mg per day to 5 every other day—without problems. I couldn't cut back on the prednisone before I came here. I've spoken my opinion and held on to it. I have more energy and a stronger frame of mind. I am not worried about what others think. Having more control over what I think and feel feels good. I'm so much better at making decisions, too. I have been taking charge."

During the two months after Helen's first visit, she began to improve. "Everything feels better," she said. "My blood pressure is lower, my blood sugar is lower, I sleep through the night now. I cut my medicines in half. My head feels great—there's just a tinge of numbness."

After four months she returned again. "I don't have pain on either side, maybe a little on the right side in my thigh, occasionally. But I don't have the sciatic [leg] pain. Just this week I have not had as much energy as before, but I have been pushing myself more and going to bed later. My sleep is great. My thumbs are a lot better, and I'm working out on the stair-stepper or walking four times a week."

Six months later I increased the potency of the homeopathic remedy because some of the joint pain and numbness returned and Helen was again waking up in the middle of the night. But four months later, when I saw her again, she reported having no joint or sciatic pain. She was sleeping peacefully through the night and feeling "better than in a long time." She was still eating well and exercising, and she was taking some of the herbs I had originally prescribed.

While preparing this chapter, I called Helen because it had been a year since I last saw her. She said, "I'm still doing well, Dr. Sullivan. You started me on the path to healing myself, and now the only time I feel bad is when I don't take care of myself. But it's nothing like before and it's temporary. I have never had the same degree of pain and sickness that I did when I first saw you. Thank you."

10

ADDICTIONS

WHAT IS AN ADDICTION?

An addiction is a compulsive and out-of-control use of a mind-altering substance or activity, despite its adverse medical, psychological, and social consequences. The substance has the ability to impair the central nervous system, liver, and kidneys, and produce withdrawal symptoms when no longer used. People usually use addictive chemicals to reduce some inner discomfort, such as anger, pain, sadness, or anxiety. The risk of addiction increases with any illness that requires prescription tranquilizers, antidepressants, or pain relievers or involves a family history of drug abuse; excess alcohol consumption; fatigue or excessive work; poverty; and psychological problems like depression and low self-esteem. There is also a physiological and mental component that drives an addicted person.

Emotionally, an addiction is a process or activity over which we are powerless. Whether it is an emotional or physiological addiction, the addiction produces a temporary pleasant mood, along with false feelings of self-confidence. The behavior of the addicted person is unpredictable and volatile. Lying, denying, and covering-up activities are common forms of behavior for an addicted person. One's perception becomes distorted, so reactions cannot be appropriate. What an addicted person says is not necessarily what he is thinking. Thus, the truth becomes distorted.

Addictions also allow people to separate themselves from their inner conflicts. We do not have to deal with the depression, pain, and confusion in our lives. But we also do not have the ability to respond to our joys and pleasures. If we are not in touch with ourselves, we cannot be in touch or intimate with anyone else. The world around us seems even more hostile, intimidating, and isolated.

In Chapter 8, I addressed the physiological and psychological problems associated with obesity. Obese and overweight people often suffer from food addiction to mask their true feelings of pain, anger, or powerlessness. The three most common food addictions are coffee, chocolate, and sugar, but Americans have many other addictions, from other drugs like alcohol, tobacco, sex, to processes like power, work, and fame.

Addictions are blind as to "race," sex, age, or color. Some addictions are more acceptable than others, simply because vast numbers of people indulge in them. Coffee, for example, is a socially acceptable addiction, partly because it is so easy to obtain and partly because so many people drink it. Most people do not consider their two or three cups a day to be an addiction, but it is.

And most people forget that caffeine is a drug. It increases one's heart rate and blood pressure and gastric acid levels. It also lowers blood sugar, stimulates the central nervous system, elevates mood, and, in large doses, creates hyperactivity and nervousness.

Patients who are trying to kick their coffee habit invariably report withdrawal symptoms, mainly irritability, nervousness, and headaches. They tell me that for the first several days after they stop drinking coffee and start on their detoxification diet, they simply do not feel well. In some cases their headaches can be as simple as minor pain; other times they are full-blown migraines.

Caffeine intake throughout the world is an estimated 70 mg per person per day. But keep in mind that in many third world countries the greatest source of caffeine—coffee—is consumed in much smaller quantities. Western countries like the United States have a higher intake of coffee. The per capita consumption of caffeine in America is 225 mg per day. More than 75 percent of caffeine ingested in America is in the form of coffee. Other forms are found in tea, chocolate, sodas, and diet pills.

When compared with the worldwide acceptance of coffee, even such hard-core, dangerous drugs as crack and cocaine carry different degrees of acceptability. The former, used more often by African-Americans than Caucasians, is less expensive and more dangerous to obtain. While cocaine use decreased from 8 million people to 4.5 million in 1993, according to the Substance Abuse and Mental Health Services

Administration, the number of crack users has remained constant over time, with an actual 5 percent increase from 1988 to 1993. In 1995, according to the National Household Survey on Drug Abuse, 1.5 million Americans are cocaine users, meaning they had used cocaine in some form within the past month. Of that number, 500,000 are crack cocaine users. According to the report, crack cocaine use was most common among young and middle-aged adult males, especially two groups: the unemployed and blacks with less than a high school education.

The distribution and use of crack cocaine carries a tougher federal penalty than cocaine powder. A first-time offender convicted in federal court of possession of 5 grams of crack will receive a mandatory prison sentence of five years. The same federal system permits probation for possessing up to 500 grams of cocaine powder.

What's wrong with this picture? The discrepancies in the severity of punishment send a message of preferential treatment and discrimination throughout society. African-Americans make up 90 percent of those sent to federal prisons for crack cocaine, even though whites make up almost two thirds of the nation's crack users. In addition, whites are more frequently tried in state court systems where the penalties are lower for the same federal offenses. Could this be just a coincidence, considering these laws follow the emergence of the crack epidemic that began with the alleged CIA covert operations in which Los Angeles street gangs were supplied with huge quantities of crack cocaine? Suddenly, tons of crack were available nationwide. And suddenly, we had the federal Controlled Substance Act, which set strict mandatory laws for possession and distribution of crack.

Another difference between crack addiction and cocaine addiction has to do with lifestyle. The behavior associated with crack makes this addiction more reproachable. Standing on street corners, meeting in alleys, robbing strangers, family members, and loved ones, having sex for money, leaving bills unpaid—these may be familiar situations for someone who is addicted to crack.

Cocaine, on the other hand, has a starkly different stereotype, one that is even respectable in some ways. Cocaine addicts may likely have a nice car and home. Maybe even a nice family. They may use the drug at a dinner or cocktail party, on a Friday night when they're relaxing with friends, or in the company of a business partner or colleague. This practice is not viewed as reprehensible, however. It is part of "life in the fast lane" in middle- and upper-class America. But the truth is, the wealthy white business executive who abuses cocaine and the poor black panhandler who's looking for a crack fix are both addicts.

Some addictions are not as taboo or dangerous as crack or heroin but are dangerous nevertheless. You don't have to be a hard-core drug user to have your life thrown upside down by addiction. Prescription drugs and alcohol are two examples of powerful addictions that have ruined lives and broken up countless families. But there are more forms of addiction. Whether it is an over-the-counter antihistamine, Valium, or a prescribed pain killer, anyone who is in the habit of abusing any form of drug is an addict.

Because it is legal and easy to obtain, alcohol is perhaps the leading contributor to serious drug addiction beyond hard-core drugs like smack and coke. Alcoholism is the result of many factors, including genetic, physiological, psychological, and social ones. And it is a costly disease. When one accounts for lost workdays, health care expenses, accidents and altercations, the price we pay as a society for the unintended effects of alcohol are enormous—upward of $120 billion a year.

The Substance Abuse and Mental Health Services Administration reported that approximately 173 million (84 percent) of the 207 million persons represented in 1993 reported alcohol use in their lifetime. Half of this number reported regular use. About 5 percent reported heavy alcohol use, which is defined as drinking five or more drinks per occasion on five or more days a month. Unfortunately, people ages eighteen to twenty-five are more likely to report heavy alcohol use, followed by those who are ages twenty-six to thirty-four. One other startling statistic from the administration revealed that 80 percent of adolescent girls use alcohol regularly. Because it is available in nearly every grocery store in the country and because laws don't prohibit the amount we drink, alcohol is one of the most accessible and socially acceptable drugs to which people become addicted.

How could we be so naive as to think that the legalization of alcohol over fifty years ago would stem the use of illegal drugs? As we have "developed" as a nation, so too have our methods of escapism from society become more sophisticated. Interestingly, between 1954 and 1975, only two drugs—cigarettes and alcohol—were used by more than 6 percent of the population who were thirty-five years old or older. But between 1986 and 1990, that same percentage of thirty-five-year-olds were abusing ten different drugs. Given the times and the pressures of life, we turned to something stronger than alcohol. And so the alcohol abuse by the children of the forties has given birth to the crack, cocaine, heroin, and prescriptive drug addicts of the nineties.

Most people do not recognize that addictions are interchangeable. People will trade one prescriptive antidepressant, antianxiety barbiturate for another, like Valium for a Xanax. The drug addict will trade heroin for methadone. The workaholic may use alcohol as an outlet. The alcoholic smokes and binges on sugar and coffee. The politician once addicted to power may shift his addiction to sex, alcohol, or money.

Addictions to the white-male-dominated system and all that it supports are killing our spirits and weakening the soul of America. As if the history of African-Americans and the current state of our communities were not enough, members of Congress recently cut budgets for major programs ranging from Head Start to Pell Grants to Medicare, while appropriating billions of dollars for B-2 bombers and nuclear submarines. And we must not forget when politicians beseeched African-American men not to rally at the capital for the Million Man March.

The issues of affirmative action and basic civil rights have been debated as if African-Americans were still considered to be only three fifths of a person. Politicians are quick to disparage the drug addictions that plague inner city neighborhoods, but they do little to amend their own abhorrent behavior. They ask the citizens of this country and the world to be responsible, while they abdicate their own responsibility. Just think back to my experience with homeless activist Milton Street, in the Introduction.

Large corporations are to blame, too. The African-American community has been a profitable arena for corporations to exploit. For instance, when have you seen a liquor store on every block in Beverly Hills or Malibu? Or how about a fast food chain restaurant every five blocks in affluent white neighborhoods? Just because they have a playground for your children does not mean the fast food these restaurants sell is good for you. The four basic food groups for Americans have become hamburgers, chicken nuggets, french fries, and sodas, loaded with hormones, tranquilizers, antibiotics, preservatives, food colorings, and caffeine. We must resist the temptations of these harmful products in order for these companies to stop invading our neighborhoods. They will only stop selling and advertising these "foods" when we stop buying them.

The chemicals in these foods add to the increased need for chemicals in our bodies. Our internal organs were not designed to process and metabolize the chemicals mentioned in Chapter 4, "Nutrition and Your Blood Type," not to mention other preservatives that contribute to hyperactivity in children. As I will discuss in the treatment section (see p. 202), there is overwhelming evidence that addictions are due more to the impairment of biochemical processes, especially the metabolism of simple carbohydrates, than to a weak will or laziness. It may be that psychological or emotional problems begin the experimentation or initiation of drug use, but you will not necessarily become addicted without the physiological component of addiction. When the body lacks proper nutrition, its metabolism is further impaired.

For example, high-fat and animal protein diets create even more problems for an individual because they disrupt the secretion of hormones from the pancreas. When this happens, the blood sugar level drops, the brain lacks necessary glucose, and our mood, motivation, and learning skills are impaired. The result is impulsive rather than rational behavior. Hypoglycemic patients have to find some substance such as alcohol, drugs, or sugar to raise the blood sugar, although only temporarily until the cycle begins again.

Biochemical imbalances are only part of the addiction story. Depression and feelings of rage also add to one's addictive habits, and the addictions of African-Americans appear to be associated with more violence than are those of white Americans, perhaps because the former have been so victimized.

Given the history of violence in America, the behavior of some African-Americans is not foreign or new. Fear and violence were embedded in the slave system. Fearful of our different language, culture, and appearance, Caucasians had to take control over black Africans and establish white male domination. Thus, the subjugation, castration, and lynching that took place during slavery were beyond cruelty. These behaviors were based on fear—fear of a myriad of behaviors that were unfamiliar and threatening.

Unfortunately, African-Americans do not have appropriate outlets to respond to this behavior. Many African-Americans are not encouraged, or even given opportunities, to release frustration, anger, or hatred in a productive way. Playing handball at the gym three times a week at 8 A.M. as the executive of a large corporation may not be an option. And while African-Americans may write movie and television scripts about violence and sex to release our anger, having them produced is a difficult task in this country. Spike Lee and John Singleton are the "exceptions" I spoke of in Chapter 5, "Stress." Nor do many African-Americans have the opportunity to pass legislation that cripples and disregards an entire ethnic group of people.

These circumstances are true for any disenfranchised group of people. A patient of European descent came to my office for treatment of hypertension. She was on Norvasc but was suffering from the unintended effects of the drug and wanted to pursue a natural approach to lowering her blood pressure. She had been on other drugs, which created even more problems, but more importantly, she wanted to support her sobriety by being drug free. "I am alcoholic but I haven't had a drink in twenty years. I was on one of the medications and I thought I was going to have a heart attack and I often lost my train of thought. It scared me."

She began telling me that she was an excitable person. She got mad and sad easily when reading the newspaper or watching the news on television. The injustice and politics of this country made her angry. Whenever people, any people, were not treated fairly she became angry. "Racism and sexism upset me tremendously. When I was drunk and experienced these situations, I would throw things and yell. Everyone on earth should have equal rights."

Judy was the youngest of five children. Her parents divorced when she was one year old. Her mother worked day and night, around the clock, to provide for her children. "I was poor and angry about it. I hated my dad and I still do. He was mean to us and to my mom. I was furious about how abusive he was to my brother. I have angry feelings toward men. They have power. They abuse women. And that makes me mad."

When her father remarried and had more children, he seldom saw Judy or her siblings. She would go to his home and get money from him, as her mother instructed her to do. "I felt humiliated because he never spoke to me—he just gave me the money in silence. I felt like I was begging."

Being poor made Judy feel inferior. She had little education and felt "stupid" and resentful. She was held back in second grade because she was not mature enough to continue. "I felt paralyzed about it, like a complete failure. I had so much shame. It's hard to dig yourself out of a hole and be all right. I could have done more with myself if I was emotionally healthy. I drank because I felt so inferior. When you are poor you are left out in the cold, alone and dependent. When you are poor, people are mean to you."

Like Judy, to alleviate inner turmoil and a sense of powerlessness, Americans turn to a substance or process that temporarily alters their mood. It begins by having a drink too often, or a joint too frequently, or a "blow" every weekend. These singular events ultimately create addictions. But over time the use of these substances exacerbates the feelings of anger, loneliness, and isolation. Eventually the use of the substance or process is necessary to reduce withdrawal symptoms (from headaches, mental confusion, and visual hallucinations to seizures) and make us feel "normal." We may be acutely aware that something is wrong, but we are likely to blame someone else, everyone else, and usually white America blames black America and vice versa. To blame means we cannot make things better and we have to wait for someone else to make it better for us. An addiction allows us to be irresponsible for our lives and our behavior.

A Case

A twenty-eight-year-old woman came into my office complaining of skin problems, insomnia and an inability to stop smoking. "I'm nervous a lot," she told me. "I just keep going. I start arguing and yelling and it feels like my head's starting to swell. I want to be able to talk without an attitude."

I asked her more about this attitude that gave her such concern.

"I'm irritable all of the time," she explained. "I get angry easily if someone picks with me and I don't want to be like that. I'm impatient, especially if things aren't organized right. I like things to be nice and neat." "Loretta" continued by saying she had terrible acne on her face and chest. She also wanted to get off of her blood pressure medication and could not stop smoking.

"I know I'm killing myself. I smoke all night long. Every two hours,

I get up and smoke. It starts at midnight and goes to five in the morning. Then I get a headache that lasts all day."

As I listened to her complain and observed her behavior in my office, I wondered if she had ever suffered from a drug or alcohol addiction. Without prompting, she eventually told me, "I started taking drugs at age twelve. I drank and smoked pot. But ever since then I've used crack regularly and been addicted to heroin. I shot heroin for four years and used cocaine for about that time."

Loretta spent much of her time as an adolescent and teenager on the street, hanging out with young boys and getting into trouble. Once she stole a school bus from the bus station because she was tired of having to walk so far home from school. Her parents did not have much to offer her. Her mother didn't work, and her father had two jobs—as a maintenance man and a truck driver for a small company. Her mother was alcoholic, but not abusive to Loretta or her siblings. Although she had five brothers and sisters, her father never married her mother, and this had bothered Loretta for the longest time.

"I just wanted them to be married—for him to come home every day and be part of the family."

When she was seven, her parents separated and Loretta had to live with her father. It was around this time that she was often out on the streets, because her father was also at work. Sometimes she would stay with her grandmother, who always had something disparaging to say about Loretta's mother.

"I didn't listen to anybody. I went to school, but I went back out the door after I got home. I raised myself. Nobody else was around."

Loretta's mother eventually married another man, who also happened to be an alcoholic. The newlyweds fought often, many times outside of the house where neighbors could witness the spectacle. Loretta was embarrassed by these outbursts and turned to the streets for solace. She began to rob and steal from others. She robbed a gas station and walked away with $1500. She and her brother robbed so frequently, she had $500 in her pocket all of the time. As she was relating these details to me, I could tell she was remorseful about these deeds. She said, despite the convenience of cash, she felt horrible for what she did and the ways in which she had harmed or frightened people.

But Loretta had her own share of personal harm. At age thirteen she was raped by an acquaintance as she was returning home from a basketball game. She didn't tell the police because she was too afraid and ashamed. She did not want to suffer the humiliation of other people knowing, so she buried the pain of this experience. At age sixteen, she had delivered her first child with a young man she had been dating for five years. This arrival of the new baby only added to her need to escape the real world and pulled her deeper into her strong heroin addiction.

She had been in jail on several occasions for stealing or assault—she had stabbed someone on more than one occasion. But the last visit to prison five years ago had lasted for four years. It was at that point she decided she would never go back to her former lifestyle. She stopped heroin cold turkey and began using other forms of drugs more frequently.

Since then her smoking had increased. She drank three cups of coffee and two diet sodas a day. Her diet consisted primarily of cheeseburgers, fried fish, and fried shrimp, with a minimal intake of water. She was irritable and impatient, and her memory and concentration were not particularly sharp. Her sleep was broken, not only by the urges to smoke but also by nightmares of being chased by someone or something trying to kill her. "I wake up scared almost nightly, until I realize it's not real."

I prescribed the remedy nux vomica 200 c because of the history of illegal drug abuse, the effects of stopping cold turkey, and the severity of her addiction to coffee, cigarettes, and diet soda. It also corresponded with her mood, her physical symptoms of fatigue, poor sleep, and decreased body temperature.

Seven months passed before I saw her again as a patient. She said that her mood and attitude were much better after the remedy, but she really was not ready to quit the coffee and cigarettes and get on the detox diet. She returned because she was ready to make some changes. Her mother was dying of cancer, which made her very distraught. She had reduced her coffee intake to one cup per day and was trying to cut back on cigarettes. I repeated her remedy and asked her to take the nux vomica in a lower potency. I also asked her to eat according to the detox diet. I gave her an herbal tincture of lobelia, valerian, passiflora, chamomile, and cayenne pepper, all of which I will discuss later in this chapter.

Again she disappeared, this time for over a year. She would periodically come into my office to purchase some herbs, but she did not come in for me to assess her condition. Nor did she ever return for a third visit to talk about her diet and blood type. But one day she came back to see me because her blood pressure medication was no longer effective in controlling her hypertension. Her blood sugar level had also become a problem.

Loretta's father had been a diabetic and her mother had suffered from a stroke several years before being diagnosed with cancer. When she came in, her blood pressure was now 146/96 and her sugar hovered in the 180s. She had stopped smoking and had reduced her coffee intake to three or four cups a week. But despite these accomplishments I could tell she was frightened about her health.

She said she had not been calm except occasionally at work. She was in a new job, which she did not like because the employees there "were racist and disorganized." The company for which she worked was six months behind on a project. Her boss began ordering her around and telling her what to do with an attitude that she did not appreciate. Loretta reminded him that she could hear, that she was a human being, and also a grown woman. Whenever he spoke to her, she could feel her blood pressure rise. This same boss had a reputation for giving more overtime to white male employees than black employees. He was also known for promoting the white males with far less experience than the black employees.

She had spent her time recently reading about natural medicine and the effects of illegal and conventional drugs on the body. Recognizing how addicted she was to a number of illegal and conventional substances, she wanted to know more about the remedies and herbs I had given her. She felt they helped her, along with her will and determination, to stop the coffee and smoking and sodas. Her sleep had improved greatly. Overall, she felt a lot healthier. She was now dreaming of adventures—winning the lottery, helping her family, and working with others.

It was clear to me that Loretta was taking her first step toward recovery: admitting she was addicted and committing herself to abstinence. After talking for a while, I decided to change her homeopathic remedy and shared with her some of the information below regarding the next steps in the recovery process, steps which involve a wholesome diet, herbs and supplements.

GENERAL DIETARY SUGGESTIONS

Conventional addiction treatment programs do not include dietary changes. So even if a person has been through a detoxification program through a hospital or private institution, it is critical that the diet also be changed. It is estimated that only 25 percent of recovered patients remain abstinent for at least three years. And some authorities say the recidivism rate is upward of 90 percent.

My patients must make a commitment to stop *all* addictive substances or behaviors, not simply their drug of choice. I explain to them that addiction is a biochemical or physiological disease. There is a problem in the way their bodies metabolize carbohydrates. As a result, the body has a desire that only addicting substances can satisfy. Refined sugar, including corn syrup products, white flour, and honey, is the main addiction. Although they are very different substances, ethyl alcohol, or ethanol, and sugar behave similarly in the body in terms of satiating the addiction. Addictions progress from this sugar addiction to other drug addictions.

Exchanging addictions will not contribute to a complete recovery. Any and all addictive substances must be eliminated so that the body has an opportunity to heal. Decreasing the amounts of some substances is not an effective approach, either. For addictive patients, I ask them for a commitment to total abstinence for a month, not just for a ten-day period as with the detoxification diet.

During this time the principles and foods listed in Chapter 4 and elsewhere throughout the book must be implemented. This includes complex carbohydrates (*not* simple carbohydrates like white rice and white flour), organic fruits and vegetables, and at least 48 ounces of distilled water a day. One must also abstain from processed foods, in any form, and especially simple sugars. Because cocaine, alcohol, and other drugs affect parts of the body like adrenal glands, liver, pancreas, and the central nervous system—the same organs that directly affect blood sugar—balancing the blood sugar is a critical step in the treatment of drug addiction. As with patients who are hypoglycemic or diabetic, I allow some protein (like fish) during the detoxification period, as amino acids stimulate the secretion of insulin and promote satiety. The patient is less likely to want more carbohydrates if protein is part of the diet.

Once the patient establishes a working relationship with a support group or therapist, and makes the commitment to abstinence for thirty days, I begin to support the patient with herbal and nutritional therapies.

HERBAL TREATMENTS
AND NUTRITIONAL SUPPLEMENTS

Herbal preparations for addictions have two basic functions: to support the liver and relieve it from abuse, and to support the nervous system and assist it in resting peacefully.

To continue the detoxification process, I prescribe large amounts of vitamin C (preferably powder form, buffered) to clean out the system. Eight thousand to 12,000 mg per day in divided doses is standard, unless that dosage creates diarrhea. Vitamin C creates very loose stools, but this is the effect I want. Vitamin C is also useful because of its antioxidant properties and its ability to stimulate the immune system by nourishing the adrenal glands. There is also evidence that ascorbic acid increases the conversion of ethanol (found in alcoholic beverages) to acetaldehyde (which is poisonous to our cells), and increases the breakdown of acetaldehyde.

The liver gets abused and impaired because of the acetaldehyde and acetate by-products that result from the breakdown of alcohol. The cells are poisoned and fatty infiltrates accumulate in the liver. There are several herbs that detoxify the liver: *Chionanthus* (fringe tree), *Taraxacum* (dandelion), *Cynara scolymus* (artichoke), and *Silybum marianum* (milk thistle). These herbs, along with other nutrients, can often be found in combination in capsule or pill form.

Fringe tree is a stimulant for the gall bladder and liver. It promotes the flow of bile into the intestine (secreted to emulsify and digest fat) and aids in draining the liver of mucus and other toxins.

Dandelion increases bile production and flow to the gall bladder. It causes contraction of the gall bladder and release of stored bile in the gall bladder itself. It is also very high in vitamins, minerals, protein, choline, and pectin. It has a vitamin A content higher than that of carrots.

The leaves of the *artichoke* have the highest concentration of substances that protect and regenerate the liver cells, while stimulating the production of bile in the liver and its transport to the gall bladder. The medicinal components of the artichoke also lower blood cholesterol and triglyceride levels.

Milk thistle actually protects the liver cells by inhibiting free radicals and leukotrienes. It acts as an antioxidant that is more powerful than vitamin E. *Silybum* components stimulate protein synthesis, which increases the production of new liver cells to replace the damaged cells.

Choline and *inositol* are nutritional supplements also used to support and detoxify the liver. Choline metabolizes and transports fat from the liver, preventing the development of a fatty liver. It is also a component of a particular fatty acid in the brain and nerve cells, and plays a role in the transmission of nerve impulses. Inositol, a form of vitamin B, also has effects on the liver. Typically, these supplements are found in combination with the herbs listed above, along with other vitamins and beet leaves.

Several herbs help reduce the insomnia and nervousness associated with withdrawal symptoms. They are: *Valeriana officinales* (valerian), *Passiflora* (passion flower), *Avena sativa* (oats) and *Chamomilla* (chamomile). While I combine these herbs in one tincture and prescribe 30–40 drops, three times a day, each of them has individual effects on the body. Valerian is a sedative that reduces blood pressure, normalizes the central nervous system, and enhances bile flow. It improves sleep quality and reduces nighttime awakenings in people who suffer from insomnia. I recommend 1–2 teaspoons of the tincture forty-five minutes before bed.

Passiflora or passion flower is primarily a depressant and reduces arterial pressure. It also acts as an antispasmodic and sedative, being particularly useful to treat the nervousness associated with a woman's menstrual cycle.

Oats have a tremendous nutritional value because of their vitamin and mineral content. Historically, they have been used for the aged and for convalescents. They are used to restore minerals and nutrients after long bouts of diarrhea. Oats are also used to recover from fatigue, because they balance the central nervous system.

Chamomile is used as a sedative and also relieves intestinal spasms and gas, heartburn, loss of appetite, and headaches.

For nicotine addictions, I add two other herbs to the ones listed above: *Lobelia inflata* (lobelia) and *Capsicum minimum* (cayenne pepper). Other names for lobelia are wild tobacco and Indian tobacco because it was smoked many years ago by Native Americans. The active ingredient in lobelia is lobeline, which is similar in its chemical structure to nicotine and has similar pharmacological actions. It stimulates receptors of the autonomic nervous system, which is then followed by depression. Lobelia increases respiration and acts as a powerful expectorant. It is therefore useful in bronchitis and asthma. Taken in toxic doses, it can have the same effects as nicotine poisoning, resulting in nausea, diarrhea, mental confusion, weakness, and faintness.

Cayenne pepper is a stimulant and a revulsant. It has been used for many years in the treatment of alcoholics.

For cocaine withdrawal, we must also support and stimulate the adrenal glands by using *Glycyrrhiza* (licorice root), *Ephedra sinica* (ephedra), and *Mentha piperita* (peppermint). Peppermint acts as a mild anesthetic on the mucous membrane lining the stomach, which counteracts nausea and vomiting, and stimulates liver and gall bladder function by increasing the release and flow of bile.

Many nutrients get depleted in an addicted person because of the effects of the drug itself, but also because people who suffer from addictions do not eat as normally or treat their bodies as well as they should. Zinc, vitamin A, carnitine, amino acids, vitamin B, magnesium, and selenium are some of the most important nutrients needed by drug-addicted people. The role of these substances and the reasons for the need to supplement them is discussed below:

- ❧ *Zinc* deficiency results from acute and chronic alcohol consumption because of decreased dietary intake and decreased absorption into the small intestine. Zinc is also excreted in the urine in higher amounts than normal in an addicted person. Low zinc levels are associated, in particular, with alcohol abuse, impaired testicular function, and cirrhosis of the liver (also alcohol related). Take 30 mg per day of the picolenate form.
- ❧ The effects of *B vitamins* are negated by drugs like alcohol and cocaine. B1 (thiamine) and B6 (pyridoxine) are especially deficient and important. A lack of B1 creates loss of appetite, fatigue, and heart and nerve disorders. A defi-

ciency of B6 creates muscular weakness, anemia, and nervousness. I prescribe a B complex vitamin (100 mg), one to three times per day.

❧ *Calcium/magnesium* deficiency is also common among drug addicts. Calcium deficiency leads to insomnia, depression, and irritability. If you are deficient in magnesium, you are prone to nervousness, tremors, and depression. Alcohol, particularly, induces excess excretion of magnesium, which continues during withdrawal. You will find calcium and magnesium in a good multimineral supplement, but if taking separately, I recommend a ratio of 1000 mg/500 mg, in divided doses.

❧ *Vitamin A* deficiency produces major complications, such as night blindness, cirrhosis of the liver, depression, fatigue, slow skin healing, testicular dysfunction, and impaired immune functions. I find that 25,000 IU per day of vitamin A is adequate for supplementation.

❧ *Carnitine* reduces free fatty acid levels in patients with liver cirrhosis, as well as triglycerides. It is synthesized from the amino acids, lysine and methionine, and vitamin C (ascorbate form), niacin, and B6. If these vitamins are deficient, then so it carnitine. Alcohol and other drugs reduce the amount of carnitine in the body, and contribute to fatty liver disease. I prescribe carnitine in 500 mg doses, two or three times a day.

❧ *Amino acids* are metabolized in the liver, and drug addiction disrupts the normal pattern of amino acids. If you suffer from depression because of withdrawal or cirrhosis, it's important to reestablish the amino acids in your body. I recommend 1 gram of glutamine per day.

EXERCISE

Exercise improves the likelihood of maintaining abstinence. Anxiety and depression are reduced through regular exercise. Also valuable as a stress reduction technique, exercise decreases the likelihood that a patient will return to drugs. Regular exercise for all blood types is essential, and for blood type A's, yoga is especially important to calm the mind and relax the nervous system.

WE HAVE TO BE VIGILANT

As with any disease, when treating addiction with natural medicine, you must *get involved.* You must take charge of your life. You must break old habits and create new ones.

We have to be more responsible. We have to be more responsible for what we put in our bodies, our minds, and our souls. We have one temple where God resides, inside of us. We have to nurture and care for it. Many of us go to church every Sunday and believe that God will make everything right once we get to heaven, as if God were separated from us on earth. What about now? What do we do now, here on earth, with God? Remember the statement from the Bible, "Thy will be done on earth as it is in heaven"? What about the God inside of you—how you are treating the spirit of the Lord?

Addiction represents a crisis in this society, a crisis of the spirit. We are hungry for the Truth. If we hope to find it in experiences that are created by something outside of ourselves, we will always be lost. We will always hopelessly be seeking what and who we already are. The image of God, made in the likeness of . . .

11

Human Immunodeficiency Virus (HIV)/ Acquired Immunodeficiency Syndrome (AIDS)

Drug addiction, specifically heroin by injection, has given rise to another long-term chronic disease: HIV/AIDS. The U.S. Department of Health and Human Services reported in 1996 that close to 150,000 people had injection-related AIDS. Of this population, 77,000, or more than half, were African-American, even though many more whites than African-Americans inject drugs. And the increasing rate of HIV infection among African-American women is due to sexual relations with IV drug users.

There are many factors involved in the interpretation of this figure. One major factor focuses on the subject of my former career, the criminal justice system. Many states make it illegal for drug users to buy needles from pharmacies, while other states also make it illegal to possess needles or any drug paraphernalia. This situation, combined with the fact that blacks who use drugs are four times more likely than whites who use drugs to be arrested for possession of cocaine or heroin, means that needles are quickly discarded in public places to avoid arrest.

By 1997 almost 582,000 people had been reported to the Centers for Disease Control with AIDS. Eighty-four percent were men, 15 percent women, and 1 percent under the age of thirteen. In 1997 the minimum estimate of people currently living with AIDS was 223,000. This estimate does not represent the larger number of people who have been diagnosed with HIV, because most people infected with the virus have not progressed to AIDS, and still more people out there have not been tested or diagnosed with HIV. In fact, the reported number of those diagnosed with HIV was 147 percent higher than the number of people living with AIDS.

Among African-Americans, the incidence of AIDS has increased dramatically. AIDS was first identified in 1981. In 1988 African-Americans represented 27 percent of all AIDS cases, 24 percent of adult male cases, 54 percent of adult female cases, and 55 percent of pediatric cases. By the beginning of 1997 an alarming 41 percent of the adults and adolescents reported with AIDS were African-American. For the first time, African-Americans are infected in greater proportion than whites. Even though declines or leveling occurred in some groups (whites, men who have sex with men, and children under the age of thirteen), increases continue among other groups such as blacks, women, and heterosexuals. The rates per 100,000 people of reported cases are near 90 for African-Americans, as opposed to 14 for Caucasian Americans! Again, as with other long-term chronic diseases, African-Americans are disproportionately represented in AIDS statistics, given the fact that blacks make up only 12 percent of the population of the United States.

This is not to say that only gays and drug users contract AIDS. Among women who have AIDS, heterosexual sex accounted for 40 percent of the cause of the infection. And 35 percent of all cases of black women are due to exposure through heterosexual contact.

I remember in 1990 when I first heard of papers that could prove HIV was developed in a laboratory in Maryland for the purpose of reducing the world population, especially people of color. I was hurt and enraged, but not from disbelief. I began to call around furiously to find out if these allegations were true and if so where I might find the documentation supporting these comments. Unfortunately, I found several books, articles, and documents that supported the fact that HIV was developed by the Central Intelligence Agency in a laboratory in their Bacteriological Warfare Division in Fort Deitrich, Maryland. European as well as American articles, books, and lectures at conferences attested to the information that the virus was put into smallpox vaccine and administered to the population on several continents, including Central Africa, South America, and Haiti.

This form of genocide is despicable. But it's happening, and no matter what position you take on the origins of the AIDS virus, we have to respond to its devastating effects on people of color. We have to forge ahead. What matters is that people of color are perceived as so dispensable and unconscious that our government would even think of, let alone carry out, such a malicious act. What matters is that we all raise our level of consciousness and create wellness for ourselves and others.

WHAT CAUSES AIDS?

There is great controversy over the question of whether AIDS is caused only by HIV or if HIV even plays a major role. In April 1996, I went to Seattle to a symposium sponsored by my alma mater, Bastyr University. During the symposium, immunologists and virologists documented the possibility that HIV was necessary but not sufficient by itself to cause AIDS. Maybe AIDS is so virulent, some of these researchers asked, because other past infections—usually many more of them than in non-AIDS patients—weaken the body and activate the HIV? Or perhaps it is lethal when there is another active virus in the person? Another idea is that, because animal viruses do not become lethal until the animals are herded together and live in close proximity, the HIV is lethal if the person is living in overcrowded conditions, like the inner city.

Another argument is that HIV is too inactive to cause AIDS, that it infects fewer cells in total than a flu virus (one in 1000 cells), and that it is too difficult to locate in an AIDS patient for it to be responsible for the damage it is said to cause. And in almost 5000 documented cases of AIDS, the HIV is not present! Because the human immunodeficiency virus is so difficult to find, doctors look for the presence of its antibodies, not the virus itself. Admittedly, it is odd that, for every other virus except HIV, the evidence of antibodies indicates that the virus is being warded off by the immune system—that the body will prevail.

There are other problems surrounding the belief that HIV causes AIDS. Since 1984, when American scientist Robert Gallo became the first researcher to claim that HIV causes AIDS, most funding to find other causes of AIDS stopped, and time and energy were devoted to understanding HIV. We suddenly put aside whatever information we had garnered from investigating the role of intravenous drug abuse, other infectious agents, and risks for AIDS resulting from suppressing the immune system, whether heterosexual or homosexual. This is particularly troubling because more funding must be directed toward other potential causes of AIDS, especially the association between AIDS and drug usage. Recall that the largest percentage of people with AIDS are men. Men consume over 80 percent of hard drugs, and it is believed that it is in this dynamic that some answers can be found regarding the cause of AIDS.

Another problem associated with the theory that HIV causes AIDS is the story behind its "discovery." A year before Dr. Gallo formally identified the virus in 1984, the virus had been discovered in France by Dr. Luc Montagnier of the Pasteur Institute. It has been revealed that the American scientist Gallo stole samples of the virus sent to Montagnier, renamed it, and wrote a fictitious paper explaining his discovery. No one checked Dr. Gallo's results. The Department of Health and Human Services later found Dr. Gallo guilty of misconduct, but he still collects millions of dollars in fees for the patent on the HIV test, which he shares with Dr. Montagnier. Today, neither gentleman believes that HIV is a deadly virus and both think that other factors are responsible for the severity of the disease associated with the virus.

I can only say I have never seen a person in my practice with AIDS who did not also have HIV. But, like other people infected for ten to fifteen years, people in my practice are well despite being diagnosed with HIV *and* AIDS (according to their T4 cell count).

I believe, as with any disease, there is still the factor of susceptibility that plays a major role in how the infection will become manifest in the body. Drug addiction and other infectious diseases, I believe, play a major role in the progression from HIV to AIDS. Every one of the patients in my practice who has been HIV-positive for a long time has never been addicted to drugs and has had few, if any, sexually transmitted diseases. Conversely, the HIV-positive patients in my practice who have passed away have all been drug addicts with at least two sexually transmitted diseases. Though they all stopped their drug of choice by the time they died, they did not stop their drug usage until they had already been diagnosed with AIDS.

WHAT IS AIDS?

Before I talk further about susceptibility, we should understand the virus and how it affects our cells. The HIV virus is composed of protein, fat, and a viral core, all of which are essential for replication. It has arms which are also made of protein that extend from the surface of the cell. These arms attach themselves to the surface of a host cell (an uninfected, normal cell). At the point of attachment is another protein called CD4. Without this protein, the HIV cannot attach itself to a normal cell.

The T-helper or T4 cells that make up part of the immune system have this particular CD4 protein on their surface. Once it is attached to the surface, with the help of several enzymes (reverse transcriptase, integrase, and protease), its outer shell dissolves and it inserts its genetic code (RNA) into the nucleus. The enzyme, reverse transcriptase, converts the HIV's RNA to DNA, and it is this DNA that is then attached to the host cell's DNA by the action of another enzyme. (The drug AZT was developed to interrupt the function of this last enzyme.)

This process changes the genetic instructions that determine the cell's functions. Essentially, the virus bursts through the protein coat of a normal cell and gradually infiltrates the bloodstream.

For some reason, the infected cells continue their normal function for a while, and in fact the immune system kills off the HIV for ten years or more (which is another reason cited for the belief that HIV does not cause AIDS by itself). At some point, however, for reasons unknown to us, pieces of the virus begin to assemble within the host cell. The third enzyme, protease, has some role in this process, but the exact steps are unknown. (This is the reason for the current use of protease inhibitors.) The pieces of the HIV push out of the infected cell and form buds. These buds of HIV destroy the host cell and then travel throughout the blood, spreading infection.

The result of this infection can be immunodeficiency and secondary infectious diseases from various organisms like tuberculosis or viruses like CMV (cytomegalovirus), EBV (Epstein-Barr virus), herpes simplex and zoster, or fungi like *Candida albicans,* and protozoa like *Pneumocystis carinii* and *Toxoplasma gondii.* Researchers who affirm that HIV by itself cannot be the cause of AIDS cite evidence that it is precisely these organisms that are already infecting the host cells and activate HIV. The T4 cell count is low before the person is diagnosed as being HIV-positive. It is peculiar that each of these organisms is responsible for a disease in and of itself. It used to be that any one of them, along with a low T4 cell count, was a definition for the diagnosis of AIDS. In 1995, however, the definition became simply a T4 count below 200.

These organisms cause various forms of pneumonia, herpes out-breaks, yeast infections, and encephalitis. Symptoms of these diseases include night sweats, weight loss, diarrhea, fatigue, fever, skin rashes, and muscle and joint pains. In more severe cases of AIDS, we see peripheral neuropathy, dementia, and malignancies (Kaposi's sarcoma, for example) along with the above symptoms.

The HIV is a retrovirus, which means that it needs reverse transcriptase (see Glossary) to reproduce its genetic code. Most viruses already have DNA when they enter the host cell and do not need an enzyme to produce themselves.

Once a virus enters the system, the body makes antibodies to the virus. In the case of the HIV, antibodies may appear from two to six months after introduction of the virus. In a small number of cases, it may take a year for the antibodies to appear. This is why it is important to be tested at these intervals, if you believe you have been exposed to the virus.

The HIV is transmitted by blood, semen (including preejaculatory fluid), vaginal secretions, and breast milk. It is not likely that the virus can be transmitted by kissing. Likewise, urine, sweat, and feces do not transmit the virus but may contain blood that could be carrying it. Thus, high-risk behavior, like using dirty syringes and needles for drug injections and having unprotected sex, put you at great risk for being susceptible to the virus. Unprotected anal sex is the highest-risk behavior because of the vast number of capillaries that are close to the surface of the anus. Unprotected vaginal sex is the second-highest-risk behavior for similar reasons. **Use a latex condom during intercourse or oral sex, not lambskin condoms, which do not protect against the virus. Women must familiarize themselves with female condoms and dental dams.**

Even if you are HIV positive, you must practice safe sex so that you reduce the risk of reinfection. Most HIV-infected people in the United States have HIV-1. Infected Africans predominantly have HIV-2. Scientists do not believe that HIV-1 and -2 have different effects on the body; they are simply different strains of the same virus. Furthermore, viruses from different individuals have been identified as aggressive and passive. The viruses isolated from people without symptoms seem to be less aggressive than viruses isolated from people with symptoms. Reinfection adds to the number of viruses in your body, which you do not want to have happen.

HIV plays a role in the cause of AIDS. We have to reduce the increasing number of people who become HIV-infected by being responsible—by discontinuing drug abuse and practicing safe sex. It is no longer a matter of what you prefer or what feels good. It is a matter of respect, responsibility, and quality of life or death. AIDS, like addictions, knows no color, sexual preference, or religious persuasion.

SUSCEPTIBILITY

Even Louis Pasteur said that the terrain is as important as the germ when he reported his "germ theory" of medicine. Unfortunately, conventional medicine chooses to ignore this important part of medicine in understanding diseases, especially AIDS. Just because you are HIV positive does not mean you will be become sick and progress to AIDS. There are people who, thirteen to fifteen years after being diagnosed, have not progressed to the diagnosis of AIDS. I have patients with a T4 cell count of less than 100 (600–800 and above is normal) *who are not sick.* But having a T4 cell count below 200 is the gauge most people use to diagnose AIDS. Thus, you do not have to be sick to have AIDS.

Some health care providers believe that everyone who has HIV will get sick and die. To date, this has not been true. I am not suggesting that people with HIV do not die from the complications from AIDS, but to have HIV is not a death sentence as some would lead you to believe. The diagnosis of being HIV positive reduces the immune function, through the stress and worry of how to live the rest of one's life, because of thoughts of suffering and death. Remember, each person is an individual, and each individual's body reacts differently to HIV.

If you have HIV, please do not allow yourself to be frightened or persuaded by a physician who has a definite idea of how long you will live, or how long before you are diagnosed with AIDS. I suggest you leave the service of that physician because he or she is doing you a grave *disservice.* These kinds of comments and predictions create susceptibility for the progression of HIV to AIDS. There is still far too much that is unknown about this disease to be definitive about its course.

As I have said throughout this book, under normal circumstances it is essential to participate in behavior that supports the health of your mind, body, and emotions. When you are infected with HIV, these life-supporting decisions become even more important. You should not associate with people—whether they are family, friends, or professional caregivers—who have rigid, negative ideas about how your life will unfold.

Blood tests also create susceptibility for HIV patients. I have seen the fear and confusion in patients' eyes when a physician announcing that their T4 cell counts have dipped below 200. Even if they are not sick, their fear is sometimes overwhelming, creating "symptoms" that have no pathological origin. The person just feels sick.

In my practice I do not focus on blood work and statistics to impress upon the patient the need for drugs or complementary medicine. Most people who come to me have already received all the statistics about their blood tests. Far too often, I have heard that their conventional doctors were quick to tell them how they had to take certain drugs to increase their T4 cell count or as a prophylactic for AIDS, but they barely mentioned the severity of the unintended effects of these drugs. Many of these same practitioners will say that you must choose between conventional and complementary medicine. This is not true.

Finally, I would like to stress how susceptibility to the conversion of HIV to AIDS can be created in other ways: the frequent use of antibiotics (common among drug users who are fighting infections from the use of dirty paraphernalia), which creates immune suppression; malnutrition; multiple concurrent infections; excessive intake of simple carbohydrates, which inhibits proper functioning of the immune system; stress-induced immune dysfunction (such as grief from loss, and feelings of isolation and depression); smoking; the use of alcohol and other drugs (especially opiates); and inadequate sleep and exercise.

DRUG THERAPY

By now most of you have heard of the drug AZT (azidothymidine), which was the first anti-AIDS drug approved for marketing in the

United States. It was prescribed for those patients with T4 cell counts below 200. Researchers began to realize after two years of AIDS patients taking this drug that it was contributing to deleterious effect on the body. Patients were developing life-threatening illnesses, they lost valuable body muscle mass and white blood cells, they suffered from anemia because of the suppression of bone marrow, not to mention the unwanted day-to-day side effects of nausea, dizziness, skin rashes, and headaches. Furthermore, researchers have discovered HIV isolates that are resistant to AZT, which means that the patient receives all of the negative side effects without any of the intended benefits. If conventional medicine is your choice, it is better to wait until this drug is absolutely necessary (T4 cells around 300). Use it for brief periods of time, one to three months, to increase the T4 cell count to a point where natural therapies can be more effective. Then discontinue its use.

Because of the resistance and toxicity problems of AZT, the next step in the conventional treatment of HIV/AIDS is a combination of AZT with ddI (dideoxyinosine), or ddC (dideooxyctidine), or simply a substitution for AZT with ddI or ddC. DdI and ddC are never to be used in combination with each other because they have similar toxicity and unintended side effects. These three drugs are the most popular, and most widely used, drugs within the scope of conventional medicine.

A more recent drug like Indinavir acts as a protease inhibitor in fighting HIV/AIDS. As mentioned previously, the enzyme protease helps activate the HIV in the cell after a certain number of years. It assists the HIV in breaking through the cell and eventually entering the bloodstream. Inhibitors are designed to interrupt the process. We do not know the long-term unintended effects of protease inhibitors, but to date it appears that some patients tolerate the drug well. In the long term, patients may incur kidney damage. And the virus may still produce mutants that are resistant. The effectiveness of these drugs is the first sign that maybe HIV does cause AIDS by itself. But it still begs the question of what activates the virus after ten to fifteen years.

I believe, in the case of HIV/AIDS, that antiviral drugs do more harm than good for the immune system. As a devil's advocate, I can suggest that, if the HIV virus was developed for the purpose of reducing the population, the associated drugs could be effective toward that same goal.

Natural therapies work alone or in combination with conventional drug therapy. There is no "cure" for AIDS in either naturopathic or conventional medicine. The goal of natural medicine is to support the immune system and to allow the body to be prepared to fight whatever it is that causes AIDS. If you are on conventional drugs, you will receive great benefit from the suggestions that follow. Natural therapies also aid in reducing toxicity and unintended effects of treatment drugs, while increasing the body's innate ability to heal itself.

While I have several patients who have HIV and who chose not to take prescription drugs, I chose to include the following case as an example of the ways that natural medicine can complement conventional medicine.

A Case

Robert, a twenty-eight-year-old African-American, came to see me several years ago because he had been diagnosed as HIV positive. He was taking several drugs to treat his condition, as well as a very powerful antifungal drug for athlete's foot. His T4 cell count when he came to see me was down to 200. He had side effects from the drugs he was taking for his HIV, and took another drug to alleviate these side effects. Over the last two years Robert had caught a cold around every six months, for which he took antibiotics for at least ten days. He had been having trouble sleeping for a period of time and he was overall depressed about his health status. When he came to me, he wanted something different than what conventional medicine was offering him.

Robert told me he had been in denial about his life. He did not want to admit his HIV diagnosis, his sexuality, and his addictions. He felt like a failure, he told me, as if he had wasted his life. "I'm afraid of failure and the future," he said, "because that is all I have ever known— failure."

Robert started drinking at age thirteen and continued to abuse alcohol later in life. He was also a coke addict in his early to mid-twenties. He stopped the cocaine abuse but still drank regularly. Guilt and shame dominated his feelings.

I learned that he had grown up masking his feelings and hiding his emotions. Pleasing others was all he wanted to do. Seldom would he speak up for himself or express to anyone what he really felt. He continued to suppress his feelings for years, and his addictions helped him mask these feelings. As Robert talked, I wondered what it was that created this need to please everyone and remain silent. But I wanted him to tell me. I did not want to probe.

His stepfather was an alcoholic and an absent role model. "I raised myself. I used to fantasize about how families did things together, because ours never did." He mentioned casually that he didn't know his father until he was fifteen. Later, Robert went to live with him. When his father realized his son was gay, he had him live with an aunt.

It was during this time that he began to get more involved in drug use. His alcoholism escalated when he dropped out of college. He had unsafe sex on several occasions with his first two lovers. His second lover died of AIDS four years into their relationship. During this time he had no support system except for the older men he was associating with. His sister was also a drug addict, while his other sister had passed away of cancer years before.

As he looked away from me and stared through my office window, he said, "I want to do something for my mom. I know she wants me to come home, but I can't be in that environment. I want to be there for my family—to pull them up, but time for wishing is over. I have to get up and do something. I have to make it happen."

He told me he used to "live for Snickers, peanut bars, and caramel chocolate candy." For a while in his life, that's all he ate, every day. Four months after being given the remedy lycopodium and completely changing his diet, he felt much better. He had more energy and was sleeping better. He was not moody or melancholy, as he had been before.

I did not see Robert for one and a half years. The next time I saw him was when he brought in his partner in a wheelchair. Carl had no strength in his extremities on the left side of his body and could barely walk. He was in an advanced stage of AIDS and was suffering from pneumonia and candida. Robert said little during this encounter, but Carl let me know that his partner was still drinking, and that it was causing a rift in their relationship.

Carl came regularly and began doing better, considering how sick he was when he came in to see me. At the end of Carl's fifth visit,

Robert promised he'd be back to continue his treatments with me. A year later he kept his promise. And he happily told me that Carl was still doing well.

"I remembered, Dr. Sullivan, how you said, 'You think this is a game you can just go play. You have to love yourself more. You have to stop drinking.' I'm in recovery, and I hear your words."

He had been in recover for a few months and was learning that he was as worthy as anyone else around him. "I am not conscious of knowing how I feel or what I want, starting with the simplicity of loving myself." He continued by telling me his T4 cell count had been around 170, and he had recently fought off an infection. But after taking several drugs, his T4 cells had risen to 210 and had remained at that level.

Despite the improved T4 count, Robert had been feeling hopeless and depressed. He was afraid of dying. Then he remembered how much better he felt after seeing me and decided to return to my care to start a regimen of herbs, diet, and homeopathic medicine.

Robert said that when he was drinking his desire to feel needed and in control was magnified. He satisfied this need by buying men for the thrill of it. And even though he didn't have sex with these men, the thought that he could do anything he wanted to them was enough of a thrill. Other times he would sell himself for sex. The idea of being paid for sex was also just as exciting.

After catching up on his life, I asked Robert very pointedly to tell me about his childhood relationship with his mother. He told me the following story. Until the age of ten, he had been afraid of his mother because she would beat him. She would use anything she could find, but usually used extension cords and rubber tubes. Sometimes she would tie him up to hit him. He remembered being left out in the cold or huddling in the shed until she came home because she never let him have a house key. And he could not go to the neighbor's home because his mother made him wait for her, no matter how long it took her to return. There were times when he would have to wait in the shed for hours.

Robert had difficulty sleeping. He often had nightmares about being chased and about people dying in accidents. "I have been in such pain, Dr. Sullivan," he said. "I don't want to keep doing it." I prescribed the remedy staphysagria 30 c daily and asked him to go back to the detoxification diet (with protein or protein powder) and prescribed herbs in order to help him withdraw from alcohol. I asked him to return in a month.

Robert kept his appointment. He reported feeling better. "I don't feel doomed like before. Occasionally, I may have a pity party, but not that often. I have work I need to do, I know. And I just need to keep on going."

Though Carl is still doing well, he and Robert decided to be just roommates. Robert had recently met someone new. In the beginning of this new relationship, Robert didn't think he was good enough for this person. But then he found himself with a new attitude and a healthy opinion about himself. "I realized I had just as much power as he did, and I focused on my power instead of his."

Our next visit was spent fine-tuning Robert's diet and discussing his herbs and nutrients.

GENERAL DIETARY SUGGESTIONS

The recommendations for HIV/AIDS patients are not that different from the recommendations for a person addicted to drugs or suffering from arthritis. Whole grains constitute the major part of the diet (45 percent), followed by vegetables (35 percent, which includes sea vegetables like wakame and kombu), legumes and fish (15 percent), nuts and seeds (5 percent, excluding peanuts). Fruits are fine, but they should be high-fiber fruits like apples, pears, and berries.

As is specified for the detoxification diet, whole grains need to be varied and should include millet, brown rice, barley, whole wheat (unless you are blood type O), oats, quinoa, kamut, spelt, and buckwheat. For all blood types, not just blood type A, you should eat as many sprouted grain breads as possible.

Vegetables should be steamed or sautéed lightly in olive, canola, or grapeseed oil. Generally three fourths of your vegetables should be cooked, and one fourth should be eaten raw. Sprouts and fresh vegetable juices are great sources of vitamins and minerals. Green leafy vegetables should be eaten and/or juiced in large quantities, especially vegetables like Swiss chard, kale, collards, broccoli, escarole, and cabbage. Garlic can be consumed up to 4 cloves per day. Seaweed, such as nori, wakame, kelp, kombu, hiziki, and dulse, should be included in the diet. (Blue-green algae, or spirulina, also provides nutrients like B12, beta carotene, and fatty acids.) Vegetables from the nightshade family (tomatoes, eggplant, potatoes, and peppers) should be kept at a minimum. Whenever possible, vegetables should be fresh and organic. Avoid canned, frozen, processed, or prepackaged vegetables.

Sea vegetables can be added to beans to improve digestion. Adzuki, kidney, pinto, black-eyed peas, red, navy, white, peas, lentils, and garbanzos are the types of beans that should be eaten regularly. When combined with grains like brown rice, quinoa, millet, etc., beans form a more complete protein. Tofu and tempeh are also forms of vegetable protein that should be consumed regularly with whole grains.

Fish is the preferred animal protein for HIV/AIDS patients, preferably poached, broiled, steamed, or baked. Salmon, halibut, haddock, orange roughy, and sardines are good choices. Cod, herring, and trout can be eaten as suggested for your blood type. Blood type A's should eat two or three small servings (4 ounces) a week. The fish, like the vegetables in your diet, should be free of chemicals. And don't forget the principles of food combinations: do not eat fish with starches or foods high in fat; eat fish or animal protein with green leafy vegetables for better digestion.

As with diabetics, I do not suggest eating large amounts of fruit. Fruit juices must be sugar-free, diluted half and half with water, and drunk slowly to avoid rapid increase of blood sugar. Sodas and artificial drinks and juices must be avoided, in addition to any forms of caffeine—coffee, black tea, and chocolate. Any simple sugar should be avoided to protect the immune system.

The detoxification diet substitutes soy milk for cow's milk and roasted grain beverages (a combination of barley, chicory, and rye) for coffee and caffeinated tea. This applies, too, if you are diagnosed with HIV/AIDS. Dandelion and, for some, wheat grass juice are also very nutritious and energizing. Combine dandelion with other green leafy vegetables for a drink rich in vitamins and minerals.

I also recommend a smoothie, which has 2 scoops of protein powder with an almond or sesame butter, yogurt, some fresh fruit, a teaspoon of maple syrup, and a teaspoon of flax oil. The proportions will need to be adjusted according to taste.

Herbal Treatments
and Nutritional Supplements

There is no cookbook therapy for HIV/AIDS patients. As with any person I treat, I am treating the person, not the HIV or AIDS. There are times when a treatment that works in one person does not produce the same results in another. Sometimes my HIV patients receive only a homeopathic remedy, a basic multiple vitamin, and one or two herbs to aid the immune system.

On the other hand, to manage AIDS, I must often treat the acute problems such as diarrhea and pneumonia. And because our knowledge of herbs and nutrients and their effects on the body is always expanding, there are constant changes in treatment protocols. Some herbs, however, have proved time and again to be useful in the treatment of HIV/ AIDS.

Please keep in mind that any natural therapy takes longer than the quick fix we are accustomed to with conventional medicine. These therapies work over time to stimulate the body's innate ability to heal itself.

Allium sativum, or garlic, has a broad-spectrum antimicrobial effect because of its sulfur-containing compounds. Its activity compares to penicillin, erythromycin, and tetracycline. Garlic also increases immune function. Take 1 clove three times a day, or 4 capsules a day.

Aloe vera has an active ingredient called acemannan, which is an immune stimulant and an antiviral. It has been shown to be active against retroviruses such as HIV. The dosage should be 800 mg per day, or 4 ounces, two times a day.

Glycyrrhiza glabra, or licorice root, is used commonly in my practice, as it has both antiviral and immune-stimulating properties. For example, it inhibits the herpes simplex virus, and it increases the activity of some white blood cells, which in turn strengthens the immune system. Again, caution should be used when taking this herb long term because of its hypertensive effects on people. I prescribe 1500 mg, three times per day, or 20 drops of fresh tincture three times per day.

Hydrastis canadensis, or goldenseal, contains a substance called berberine that has a broad range of antibacterial and microbial activity. It also inhibits excess candida growth, a common side effect of excessive antibiotic use, and soothes the mucous membranes of the digestive and respiratory tracts (in cases of diarrhea and pneumonia, respectively). Goldenseal has tremendous benefits to one's immune system by activating white blood cells responsible for destroying bacteria, viruses, fungi, and tumor cells. During cold and flu season I use this plant regularly in my practice. I prescribe 20 drops three times a day, or 1500 mg a day in divided doses.

Hypericum perforatum, or St. John's wort, has been shown to be antiviral because of its active constituent, hypericin. It is particularly effective against herpes I and II, and has been shown to stop the entry of HIV into host cells. This herb should be taken with meals. Recommended dosage is 2 to 10 mg of hypericin per day, or 30 drops of the tincture, three times a day.

Lomatium species (leptotania) or *Ligusticum porteri* (osha root) are plants I use because they have antiviral properties. Studies have shown that lomatium inhibits the replication of HIV.

Mormodica charantia, or bitter melon, has been known to increase T4 cells and energy over time. As the name suggests, it is a very bitter-tasting herb. For this reason, and so that the protein in bitter melon is not broken down by the stomach acids, I recommend a retention enema. Through this method, the proteins can be absorbed directly into the bloodstream through the colon and large intestine.

Maitake mushrooms are also used to stimulate immune activity by producing more white blood cells and increasing T4 cells. These mushrooms also have antitumor benefits and have been used for thousands of years in China and Japan. I recommend 3 capsules, three times a day.

There are other antiviral herbs that have been used in the treatment of HIV/AIDS, but it is beyond the scope of this book to name them all. There are, however, two other plants that show some promise for treatment: *Dionaea muscipula,* or Venus's-flytrap or carnivora, and grapefruit seed extract. They are used to increase T4 cells and kill different microorganisms, respectively.

For recently diagnosed HIV patients, I use a combination of *echinacea* and *engystol* in low-potency homeopathic liquid form. Ideally, these substances should be injected, but I administer it to the patient in distilled water. I have been using this protocol ever since I read an article in the Internal Medicine World Report (April 1991) regarding the efficiency of the substances in preventing HIV patients from becoming AIDS patients. With the exception of one patient under my supervision, my HIV patients have not been diagnosed with AIDS. Of course, this is not the only treatment I use, but in combination with the other herbs and diet, this seems to be effective. A word of caution: echinacea in its whole form (tincture, dried herb, extracts, capsules, etc.) is not to be used chronically for people with HIV/AIDS, but rather only as part of an acute treatment.

The nutritional supplements for the treatment of HIV/AIDS are a variety of products. By now you know that every one of my patients is asked to take a basic multiple vitamin and mineral supplement. These supplements should be without fillers, binders, or preservatives to guard against hypersensitivity reactions and to insure maximum absorption. In addition to the supplements, there are other essential nutrients for the HIV/AIDS patient: *beta carotene* (300,000 IU in divided doses), *vitamin C* (1 gram every two hours to begin treatment) with *flavonoids* (500 mg, three times per day), *vitamin B* complex (50–100 mg), especially *B12* (1000 mcg injected into the muscle, once a week), *flax* or *cod liver oil* (1 tablespoon, two times per day), *coenzyme Q 10* (50 mg, three times a day), *quercetin* (2 capsules, two times per day) and *zinc* (15–30 mg per day). Coenzyme Q10, specifically, provides energy to the tissues and cells of the immune system and increases some of the cells of the immune system. Quercetin is an inhibitor of the reverse transcriptase and integrase enzyme.

Antioxidants are also important in the treatment of HIV/AIDS, because they assist in protecting the cells from damage by free radical oxygen compounds (or oxygen-missing electrons). Antioxidants make free radicals more stable by adding more electrons. Some examples of free radical scavengers, or antioxidants, are *pycnogenol, N-acetylcysteine, beta carotene, vitamins C* and *E* (400 to 800 IU per day), *selenium* (200 mcg), *zinc* and *flavonoids*. These nutrients are referred to throughout the book, with the exception of pycnogenol and N-acetylcysteine.

Pycnogenol is a flavonoid that almost all people easily assimilate. It is extracted from maritime pine trees and is also found in grape seeds. Grape seed pycnogenol extract is more effective than pine tree extract, though both are acceptable and useful sources. A daily dose of 50 mg is recommended for non-HIV patients, and 150 to 300 mg is recommended for HIV/AIDS patients.

N-acetylcysteine reduces the HIV-1 replication and is necessary for the synthesis of glutathione, the main antioxidant protecting the mitochondria—the cells that generate energy from foods. The recommended dosage for N-acetylcysteine is 2000 mg per day.

Some of the more acute heath concerns associated with HIV/AIDS actually have common natural remedies: gastrointestinal nutrient absorption and pneumonia can be treated with remedies like acidophilus, amino acids, grapefruit seed extract, rosemary, psyllium seed husks, oat bran, and digestive enzymes. Herbs for respiratory problems associated with *pneumocystis carinii* pneumonia, for example, include *aspidosperma, elecampane, glycyrrhiza, hydrastis,* and *sanguinaria* to be taken in conjunction with whatever immune stimulant you are taking.

As a naturopathic physician, I believe that homeopathic and herbal medicine, diet and nutrients are indeed the foundation for one to rebuild physical vitality and immunity. But I would be remiss in my obligation as a healer if I did not stress the necessity of individual and group psychotherapy, meditation, affirmations, and spiritual practices like yoga, tai chi, or qi gong. And this is especially true for HIV patients.

I recommend the following books to my patients to aid in their psycho/emotional healing:

You Can Heal Your Life, by Louise Hay
You Can't Afford the Luxury of a Negative Thought, by John Roger and Peter McWilliams
A Course in Miracles, from the Foundation for Inner Peace
A Return to Love and *Illuminata,* by Marianne Williamson
The Tibetan Book of Living and Dying, by Sogyal Rinpoche
Acts of Faith and *Tapping the Power Within,* by Iyanla Vanzant

For a more general book about HIV and AIDS, I recommend, *No Time to Wait: A Complete Guide to Treating, Managing, and Living With HIV Infection,* by Nick Siano.

A Final Word About AIDS

Clearly, many more Americans and especially African-Americans die from heart disease and cancer than from AIDS. Consider AIDS a warning, a signal that we are a society burdened by addictions, environmental and dietary stress and toxins, and our own inability or unwillingness to love. I believe all things come from God. AIDS is an opportunity to heal the separation and isolation that had permeated our society long before the virus was identified. There are probably few among us who do not know someone directly or who do not know someone who knows someone who has HIV or AIDS. We are all affected, as individuals and as a society. God is demanding that we love each other or perish in our disease of judgment and criticism.

Within the black community, being a leper is more acceptable than being gay, especially for young black men. There is no greater stigma in the African-American community than male homosexuality. The reproach that accompanies this sexual persuasion is crippling (for those who are judges and those who judge). African-American gay men, often filled with self-hatred and disparagement, have enormous challenges to feel worthy. Discrimination for a gay African-American male is based on sexual preference *and* color.

Hatred of any part of yourself is a spiritual crime because we are all God's creation. The penalty is continued self-denial and abnegation. Black gay men, especially, have been taught the power of hate and fear, but certainly not the power of love.

Whenever I have been in a state of confusion and felt alone, it has been because I have separated myself from God. In order to heal, I have had to be more open to the Truth. I have been more willing to be vulnerable (open) to receive whatever Spirit brings forward for me to look at about myself and personality. I have had to surrender my irritations and disappointments to Spirit, by opening up to the God inside of me—the part that knows—and asking to be more loving. By sitting down with myself *every day* to listen to my God self, I have learned to expand when I want to withdraw and contract. I have learned to just keep putting the next foot forward. I have experienced choosing to let God out because keeping the Spirit in me, tucked away and hiding, is too painful. I have experienced God is love.

I have had to have faith and trust, not in someone or something else but in the knowing that God has not taken me this far to let me down. I will be taken care of, always. I know the universe is here to support me; that God gives me everything I need. Even if I do not like it, the key is to learn from it, especially if I do not like it. I have had to let go of my fears.

When I have felt alone and confused, I have had to put aside my judgment to get out of my own way, in order to focus on loving. In my life, as in everyone's, it has been important to stop holding on to hurt feelings or anger and forgive myself for judging another as wrong. I have had to recognize that people react out of hurt feelings and fear, very often unrelated to the moment and their interaction with me. They are reacting through a filter that has years of pain and fear woven into it. It does not mean I have allowed people to treat me any way they want. It means I have forgiven my judgment of them, loved them, and chosen not to participate with them anymore.

When we feel confused and isolated, in order to survive ultimately, each of us must make our own choices about how we are going to be kind to ourselves and show ourselves that we love ourselves. That is why we are here together—to aid each other in that process. To interact with one another so that we each know the depth of loving within us. Love the person who hurts your feelings because they give you an opportunity to be more loving, to reach deeper into the awareness that we are all one and that you are special just as you are. They give you an opportunity to support and love yourself more. You do not have to be their friend, you just have to love them. Maybe through the state of confusion and isolation, which is symbolized through the growing numbers of AIDS victims and judgments against them, we as a society can open to the Truth. I hope we can learn and grow with that Truth and bring heaven and earth together, bringing an end to the pain and suffering around us. Hate can only be healed by loving.

Thoughts are powerful. We are all angels, I believe, who chose to enter the world to have experiences so that we can learn the lessons we need in order to go "Home" and stay "Home." Or, stated another way, to have everlasting life. We cannot have those experiences in any other form besides that of human flesh. It is important to have interactions with others in order to teach us how to love ourselves and humankind. To fall in love with yourself deeply is the goal. Love others from the overflow. Forgive yourself for your issues and imperfections. Be gentle with yourself and recognize that you have done nothing wrong. Laugh more and be spontaneous.

Support yourself by doing things that help you to heal. Believe in your treatments and your healing. Do not give up or be impatient. HIV is not a death sentence but a catalyst to change your life.

12

CANCER

WHAT IS CANCER?

Every disease begins at a cellular level. The cells make up organs, so it is important to nourish the cells of our bodies. It is also important that cells eliminate waste properly. When cells do not receive proper nutrition (because of the consumption of too much fat, or because foods are cooked in oils at very high temperatures that change the structure of the cell wall) or do not eliminate toxins effectively the cells become diseased. Once the cell is diseased it has the incorrect genetic information to perform its appropriate function. Once this cell reproduces into other cells a tumor forms, composed of these cells. The body's defenses may be able to destroy these foreign cells or at least keep the tumor localized. Normal cells know how many to reproduce and when that reproduction should occur. Malignant, or cancer, cells seem to have minds of their own, as they produce rapidly and without any pattern. In some cases the cells are so disorganized that they break away from the original tumor and travel to other parts of the body. This is known as metastasis.

Researchers have noted the cause of cancer to be multifactorial; specifically that genetics, radiation, and carcinogenic agents (pesticides, asbestos, etc.) all play a role in causing cancer. More recently, mainstream medicine has added diet to the list. And most recently, some allopathic physicians are now recognizing the role of stress as one of the factors affecting the cause of cancer. As a naturopath, I believe diet and stress speak directly to why our bodies do not protect against the development of cancer. Or, stated differently, it is diet and mental and emotional stress that decrease the ability of our immune systems to function effectively against the production of cancer cells once our normal cells are damaged by carcinogenic agents or radiation. Strengthening your immune system and getting screening tests are essential elements of the fight against cancer.

Prevention Is the Best Cure

Similar to HIV/AIDS, cancer can be a catalyst for making changes in one's life. But too often people make these changes *after* they are diagnosed with the disease. What if we could change our lives before we developed a long-term chronic disease? What if we were more involved in the primary prevention of our illnesses?

Prevention of any disease is important, but this is especially true of cancer. There is no cure for advanced stages of cancer, and conventional cures for early stages are very toxic. Screening tests are absolutely essential. Women over fifty must receive regular gynecological and mammographic exams and men over forty must receive regular prostate examinations. But these tests are secondary, not primary, steps toward prevention. We must do much more than take tests to reduce the risk of any form of cancer.

Primary prevention means receiving negative gynecological, mammographic and prostate test results because you have taken the preventive measures to eliminate the risks of cancer. Primary prevention means you are eating whole foods, without chemicals, you have reduced or eliminated drugs like nicotine, caffeine, alcohol, you have begun to exercise regularly, and you take supplements to strengthen and protect your body.

As I discussed in Chapter 4, "Nutrition and Your Blood Type," diet is the first step toward achieving healthiness and is usually the first stumbling block on one's journey toward the primary prevention of cancer. The American Cancer Society states that up to one third of the 560,000 cancer deaths in 1997 were related to poor nutrition. The amount of junk food we consume contributes to these numbers. I have some patients who drink over 150 cans of soda a month, and others who eat over a dozen doughnuts a week. How do we expect a body to function effectively without proper nutrition and with the subsequent waste that remains in the system after consuming so much junk food?

When one considers how often we consume meat laced with tranquilizers, hormones, and antibiotics, vegetables covered in chemicals
and pesticides; when we think about the pollution in the air we breathe
and water we drink; when we think about the drugs and alcohol we
indulge in, both recreational and prescribed, it is a wonder that we do
not have even higher rates of cancer in this country.

DIAGNOSIS AND RISK FACTORS

Diet and personal habits are part of the story. Diagnosis is another. For
a time, researchers tried to link cancer to genetics as a reason for the
high incidence of cancer among black people. But now we know victims
of cancer are racially disproportionate because of environmental, occu-
pational, and economic factors. One in eight women in the United
States between the ages of one and eighty-five has a lifetime risk of
getting breast cancer. While Caucasian women have a higher incidence
of breast cancer than African-American women, African-Americans are
twice as likely to die of it than Caucasian Americans. This is due in part
because African-Americans are diagnosed at more advanced stages of
the disease. Another reason is that African-American women are more
likely to be overweight or obese than white women, and women who
are obese are more likely to die from breast cancer. There are also other
risk categories for African-American women that put them at greater
risk for cancer. For instance, women who have no insurance have 2.3
times higher risk of death from breast cancer than women with private
insurance. Women who were divorced, separated, or never married have
increased risk of death. And finally, women who are childless or menopausal, women with a family history of breast cancer, and women who
consume excessive amounts of alcohol and sugar all run greater risks of
breast cancer.

African-American men have a higher overall cancer rate than any
other racial or ethnic group in America. African-American men have
higher incidence rates of cancers of the prostate, lung, and oral cavity
than any other ethnic group. They also have the world's highest
chance of developing prostate cancer, along with the highest mortality
rate from this disease. White men have a higher five-year survival
rate than African-American men. This may relate to the fact that

higher animal fat consumption may be associated with a higher risk for prostate cancer, as it is for breast cancer, and that African-American men typically consume more animal fat than their white counterparts.

In addition to the dangers of poor diet, we know that all cancers caused by cigarette smoking and heavy alcohol use could be prevented completely. Smokers are ten times more likely than nonsmokers to develop lung cancer. And even breathing secondhand smoke puts you at greater risk for cancer. About 35 percent of African-American men and 22 percent of African-American women smoke. The American Cancer Society estimates that in 1997 about 174,000 cancer deaths were caused by tobacco use, and another 19,000 cancer deaths by alcohol abuse.

If we continue to avoid doctors because of all of the variables I mentioned in the beginning of the book—including lack of insurance—primary prevention becomes even more critical for our fight against cancer. We cannot afford *not* to take preventive steps *and* get examinations that may reduce the risk of early death.

PROSTATE CANCER

Although it is beyond the scope of this chapter to discuss all of the various forms of cancer that affect Americans, prostate cancer is becoming an increasingly important issue because it is the second leading cause of cancer death among African-American men, behind lung cancer. I strongly urge all African-American men over forty in my practice to have a prostate examination yearly, especially if they have a family history of cancer, if they come in contact with chemicals or toxic waste on a regular basis, or if they smoke or drink excessively. Also, men who have had a vasectomy are believed to have a greater risk of prostate cancer. A prostate examination includes a routine rectal examination and blood work.

Male patients who believe they may have prostate cancer may suffer a range of urinary problems, from frequent urination to an inability to urinate. The person may experience pain with urination or ejaculation and rectal pain during bowel movements. Pain in the back legs and hips may also indicate prostate problems. But any or all of these conditions can also be signs of benign prostatic hyperplasia, a noncancerous condition of the prostate.

If diagnosed in the early stages, prostate cancer can be treated and cured in most cases. However, most black men do not want to go through the discomfort of a rectal exam. A doctor who feels something suspicious in the rectum will usually order a biopsy of the area. If the biopsy tests positive for cancer, the doctor will then order more tests, including X-rays and blood work to determine whether the condition has spread to other parts of the body. If the tumor is small and localized, surgery alone may be sufficient to remove it. If the patient is older, the doctor may have to perform radiation treatment.

A 1993 report in the *Journal of the American Medical Association* states that prostatectomy (the removal of all or part of the cancerous prostate gland) and radiation may not be the best treatment for prostate cancer. The report states that it may be better for the patient to monitor the tumor's progress and withhold treatment until absolutely necessary. Naturopaths, believing this wait-and-see approach may be the best alternative for prostate patients, will prescribe natural remedies in the meantime. (See p. 242, "Herbal Treatments and Nutritional Supplements.") If not diagnosed or treated in time, however, prostate cancer can spread to any organ in the body. The most common sites for its spread are the bones and lymph nodes. With such a diagnosis, chemotherapy or hormonal therapy is absolutely necessary.

BREAST CANCER

Breast cancer has been a popular and controversial topic of discussion in recent years. Studies arguing the benefits of mammograms and the link between breast cancer and breast implants have earned this subject considerable media attention and public concern. For these reasons, and for the fact that most of my cancer patients who come into my office suffer from breast cancer, I am devoting a larger section of this chapter to this one form of cancer.

Each of us must do self breast examinations or have a breast examination performed by a professional, regularly. If you find a lump, it may be fibrocystic breast disease (usually painful breast lumps that change with your menstrual cycle) or possibly cancer. Do not hesitate to get a definite diagnosis. Being proactive can save your life. Ask questions. Do not let your physician intimidate you or talk over your head. Ask him or her to explain whatever you do not understand. Don't be shy. It is *your* breast and *your* life. The following information will assist you in understanding the process of diagnosing and treating cancer.

At Bastyr University, I learned that cancerous lumps were usually hard, immovable, and associated with discoloration and dimpling of the skin. This is not always the case. So if you have any doubt about a lump in your breast, check it out. Normally I do not recommend a mammogram until age fifty, but if you have a suspicious breast lump you should have one. If the mammogram does not give you definitive results, you should request a diagnostic ultrasound examination (especially if you are premenopausal), which can tell you whether or not the lump is hollow or solid. The former type of lump is indicative of a cyst. The latter is not necessarily cancerous, but more investigation is needed to determine just what type of lump it is—benign or malignant (cancerous).

If you still do not have definitive results from these tests, it is likely that your physician will recommend a biopsy—removal and examination of tissue from the body, in this case some of the cells of the lump. Aspiration or needle biopsy is the least invasive. It involves a local anesthetic after which a needle is inserted into the tumor and some fluid or cells are removed. Once the cells are removed, a pathologist determines if they are cancerous. Be aware that doctors unfamiliar with this procedure may not extract any cancerous cells during the procedure. This means the pathologist will not diagnose the breast cancer even though cancerous cells may exist. So be sure you trust your doctor and his or her experience with biopsies.

The other possibility for examination is a surgical biopsy or lumpectomy. This procedure removes the tumor and surrounding healthy tissue. After performing a lumpectomy, the surgeon will suggest that some of the lymph nodes from the axilla (armpit) of the affected side be removed and examined. If cancer has spread to the nodes in the armpit on the same side as the affected breast, the prognosis is worse than if the cancer were isolated within the breast. But it is by no means a death sentence.

The degree of nodal involvement gives you an indication of your prognosis or chances of survival. Thus, some people do not want to know their nodal results. As with HIV and T4 cell counts, you may not want to know the extent of the cancer in your body, as it may create more negative thought processes and decrease your will to fight. Generally, half of all breast cancer patients have nodal involvement and half do not.* Removing all of the lymph nodes will obviously reduce the likelihood of cancer reappearing in that part of the body, but it does not necessarily reduce the likelihood that cancer will not appear in the breast again or somewhere else in the body. It is also not clear that removing all of the nodes extends life expectancy. The complications of lymph node removal include pain, numbness, and tremendous swelling of the affected arm.

However, if you are premenopausal, knowing the status of the lymph nodes is important because chemotherapy may be necessary to treat your lymph nodes. Chemotherapy does not provide as much benefit if you are postmenopausal, and very questionable benefit if your lymph nodes are not involved or if the tumor is less than one centimeter in diameter.

The degree of nodal involvement and tumor size determine the "stage" of the cancer. If your tumor is two centimeters or less in diameter, without nodal involvement, you have Stage I cancer. If your tumor is two to five centimeters, with limited or no nodal involvement, you have Stage II cancer. Stage I and II are early-stage cancers.

The treatment of choice for many years was radical mastectomy for most cases of breast cancer. This procedure removes the breast, chest muscle, and the adjacent lymph nodes. A critical review of this procedure was released in the *Journal of the American Medical Association* over thirty years ago but was virtually ignored by physicians and surgeons. After much research in the 1970s and 1980s, many surgeons agreed that this method of treatment is no more effective than less invasive techniques. Since that time, radical mastectomy has been replaced with a "modified radical" procedure, which involves removal of the breast and lymph nodes or just a "simple mastectomy," which is removal of the breast only.

One of my teachers at Bastyr University, Dr. Steve Austin, has written a very informative book, *Breast Cancer: What You Should Know (But May Not Be Told) About Prevention, Diagnosis and Treatment.* He re-

*Austin and Hitchcock, *Breast Cancer,* p. 19.

views many studies and concludes that these studies comparing lumpectomy alone, lumpectomy with radiation, and mastectomy have shown that the survival rates are no different among these treatment procedures. However, the recurrence of breast cancer is higher in women who have only a lumpectomy without radiation treatment. You should be given a choice if you have early-stage cancer, though too often the only choice offered to patients is a modified mastectomy. It has been shown that a lumpectomy is just as effective as a mastectomy, even when the tumor size is four centimeters or greater.*

Doctors usually include radiation treatment with a lumpectomy, but if you have had lung disease or previous irradiation, you should not receive radiation treatment. Radiation may also damage the ribs, the lungs, nerves that supply the arm and the breast, and always decreases energy for a long period of time. The younger you are when the radiation is performed, the more likely it is to increase your risk of developing another cancer, since radiation is carcinogenic. The treatments require frequent visits to the doctor's office, which can be depressing in and of itself.

Dr. Austin also writes that researchers around the world have been investigating this issue of radiation accompanying lumpectomy. Women with small tumors—less than a centimeter in diameter—are good candidates for abstaining from radiation without running high risks of recurring breast cancer. While women over seventy are good candidates for omitting radiation, those in their thirties and early forties (before age forty-five) have a relatively higher risk of recurrence of breast cancer and should strongly consider this procedure. I find this to be consistent with the women in my practice and advise them accordingly.

You do have a choice about surgery. The chance of survival is no different whether you have a lumpectomy or a mastectomy. But I know from my patients that many doctors will not tell you this. They will tell you to remove the entire breast. Fortunately, there are now state laws that require doctors to tell patients about their options. In those states fewer mastectomies than lumpectomies are performed. For example, more mastectomies are performed in the South than in the Northeast.

---

*F. Habibollahi and I. S. Fentiman, "Breast Conservation Techniques for Early Breast Cancer," *Cancer Treatment Review,* 1989; 16: 177–91.

Before making any decisions, read! The books I recommend are: the aforementioned *Breast Cancer: What You Should Know (But May Not Be Told) About Prevention, Diagnosis and Treatment,* by Steve Austin, N. D., and Cathy Hitchcock, M.S.W., and *Dr. Susan Love's Breast Book.*

While it is beyond the scope of this chapter to discuss all of the treatments and protocols relative to breast cancer, it is necessary for me to include a brief discussion about chemotherapy. Currently, chemotherapy is suggested as an additional treatment in early-stage cancer. I believe, like the radical mastectomy, that this treatment is excessive in most instances. But others argue that women with breast cancer have what is called micrometastasis, or small pockets of cancer, that may be removed with chemotherapy. So in theory, because doctors cannot speak for every individual case, medical doctors believe most women should receive chemotherapy.

Even though we know that the spread of breast cancer is not due solely to the breast tumor, and that cancer affects the whole body and all the levels of the body, conventional medicine still treats it as a localized disease. As a naturopath, I believe in the body's ability to fight cancer, given the proper support and intervention. Supporting the body, then, and not destroying it unnecessarily, is the key. There is no proof that chemotherapy is the best treatment for micrometastasis.

The research on the value or success of chemotherapy does not factor in the quality of the woman's life, only the fact that she is still "alive." It does not consider the nausea, vomiting, baldness, low self-esteem, inability to perform everyday tasks and responsibilities, loss of sex drive, and family and marital problems. But while chemotherapy may decrease the chance of a recurrence of breast cancer, it does not decrease the risk of it occurring in bone, liver, or lung, which are usually more fatal.*

There are many American physicians and researchers (but not enough) who agree with European colleagues that chemotherapy in early-stage cancer is unnecessary in women whose lymph nodes are negative for cancer cells and whose risk of recurrence is low. Almost 70 percent of patients whose lymph nodes are cancer-free are cured with-

Lancet 1994; 343: 377–81.

out chemotherapy, and most of those patients who would ultimately die from breast cancer will not be cured by chemotherapy.*

More research needs to be done on what constitutes low risk. However, those whose tumor is one centimeter or less, and who have non-invasive cancer that is designated by the pathologist as tubular, colloid, mucinous, or papillary have been determined as low risk. Those with tumors between one and two centimeters with ER-positive status (estrogen receptors on breast cancer cells; if positive, there is a better prognosis) and a good grade are also low risk.†

For those who have no cancer in the lymph nodes but are not at low risk, there are other options: chemotherapy or surgical removal of the ovaries. The prestigious medical journal *Lancet* published several studies in 1992 that present removal of the ovaries as an alternative to chemotherapy especially for postmenopausal women in their forties. It is clear that premenopausal women benefit more from chemotherapy than postmenopausal women who have positive lymph nodes. Specifically, these studies indicate that premenopausal women who lost their menstrual cycle as a result of the chemo have greater survival rates.

When the menstrual cycle is stopped estrogen production decreases. Estrogen promotes cancer growth. The effectiveness of chemotherapy is due in part to the destruction of ovarian function and their ability to produce estrogen. Ovarian ablation, as it is called, for women under fifty was just as effective as chemotherapy, especially if the ER status was high (greater than 20). Yes, there are problems with loss of ovarian function too, like hot flashes, vaginal dryness, and greater risk for osteoporosis. But loss of function is loss of function. It does not matter what is the cause. Given the side effects of chemotherapy mentioned earlier, it would be wise to consider ovarian surgery as an option to chemotherapy.

Tamoxifen is the only other conventional treatment I want to discuss. Postmenopausal women who are ER-positive with lymph node involvement receive greater benefit than women who are premenopausal or whose nodes have no cancer. Tamoxifen was developed as a contraceptive to bind to estrogen receptors and thus interfere with estrogen.

*New England Journal of Medicine 1992; 326: 1774–75
†Journal of the National Cancer Institute 1992; 84: 1479–85.

Unintended effects of this drug include hot flashes, vaginal dryness, menstrual irregularity and, in a small number of women, uterine cancer if it is taken for over two years.

These choices and decisions regarding treatment are difficult ones. But they must be made. Do not wait for God to heal you as some of my patients choose to do. In my experience, God has to know that you are doing your part in this healing process. When you put your foot forward God will meet your halfway. Review as much information as possible. Other books I would recommend are *The Politics of Cancer* by Samuel Epstein and *Love, Medicine and Miracles* by Bernie Siegel, M.D.

We cannot forget the psycho/emotional state of so many cancer patients that results from one form of abuse or another. Many of the women I see with cancer have histories of abandonment, abuse, feelings of worthlessness, powerlessness, anger, fear, and repression. Too often I hear statements like: "I've lived my life reacting to fear and anger inside." "I've always felt so small and angry." "I've always had to justify my worth and reason for existing." After hearing this kind of testimony from so many of my patients over the years, the cause of this disease is easier for me to understand, especially when I consider what cancer really is: the destructive, uncontrolled growth and spread of abnormal cells—cells that eat away at the normal cells of the body, just as anger and pain eat away at the psyche. Given all of the addictions, anger, hatred, and pain in America, is it any wonder we Americans have the highest cancer rate of any people on the planet?

Recently a forty-year-old Caucasian woman with breast cancer came to my office after undergoing three rounds of chemotherapy and a mastectomy even though she had lymph node involvement! Paula was frequently ill even before she started the chemotherapy. She was in an unhappy marriage. Her husband was not abusive (she had had enough abusive men in her life), but she no longer loved him and was often disgusted by his hedonistic behavior. She knew he loved her but "the way he loves me is not what I need."

From early adolescence to adulthood, she had felt lonely, angry, misunderstood, and unsupported. She said, crying, "I've had so much pain and despair. There's been no support for who I am. I have a history of abandonment." Neither parent was affectionate or supportive of her: her mother was cold and her father nasty and verbally abusive. Paula felt very alone and yet had to be responsible for raising her siblings after her parents were divorced at an early age. Her mother left the children and her father had custody. Paula was responsible for everything—the cooking, cleaning, grocery shopping, laundry, etc. "I was confused and ashamed. My life was chaotic and I was living in darkness. Every page of my diary from that time in my life says 'Help.' "

After a series of abusive relationships she married her husband because "he wanted to marry me and I wanted to marry. It made logical sense." Now, having been diagnosed with breast cancer four months ago after a routine exam, she was haggard-looking and fatigued, and suffered from all of the unintended side effects of chemotherapy—the nausea, vomiting, baldness, dizziness, and loss of sex drive. She also had mouth sores, profuse night sweats and joint pains. Again she cried as she said, "I've been given this life and I feel I blew it; I haven't dealt with it well at all. I feel I gave myself cancer because of the pain inside of me." I prescribed the remedy carbo animalis in a 12 c potency, three times a day, and subsequently changed her diet and added nutritional and herbal supplements that I will discuss later in this chapter.

After a month of taking the remedy, changing her diet and adding supplements Paula's appetite increased and she was capable of eating more easily despite another round of chemotherapy. The changes I had prescribed assisted her through the treatments and, rather than being sick, she felt much better after taking them. She had no mouth sores or joint pains. She was not as discouraged or weary. She was making plans for the rest of her life rather than letting life happen to her. Paula was no longer fearful of death or of being alone.

She said something else to me during our first visit, similar to what I hear from so many other breast cancer patients: "I love being a mother. I love nurturing. I loved breast feeding. It makes me feel soft and connected. It's as if you can see all the goodness you have being brought up in front of you."

Breasts symbolize nurturing and abundance. It is fascinating to think of this in relation to how much women are expected to bear and to give, and how many people we are supposed to nurture throughout our lifetime. Often without anything left for ourselves, we continue to give and feel guilty when we do not give enough. It's a miracle the cancer incidence is not higher! For many women, the soil or terrain for a degenerative disease like cancer is fertile.

ANOTHER CASE

"I have always been a serious person. I've always taken on a lot of responsibility for others. I lived my life feeling a lot was expected of me, and I've misused my body in the process. It's important to help others and remember where you come from. But you can do that and not hold on to where you've come from. You can do that and still shine. Some choices I made, I made because I thought I shouldn't shine." After this statement, Janice paused for a long time. Then, as she let out a deep sigh, she said, "I've never told anybody that before. There are so many things I've never said before."

Eventually during our meeting Janice, a middle-aged African-American woman, revealed that her father was alcoholic and beat her mother badly. As a result, Janice was nervous and frightened for most of her childhood. She was in tears when she told me that one night her father pulled a gun on her brothers, who were trying to restrain him from beating their mother. "I was so scared, I just cried and cried and begged him not to shoot them."

Throughout her life Janice continued to be afraid because of her abusive relationships. Although she was a good student, she dropped out of school at age eighteen because she was pregnant. She had been with her boyfriend since junior high school. He would shout at her and criticize her constantly. "I never felt worthy because of this relationship and because I didn't do what I was supposed to do. I didn't do what was expected of me by my parents." Janice had subsequently married and divorced another man.

For the last six years Janice had been abused by her live-in boyfriend. They had been together for sixteen years, but only in the last six years had he begun to physically and verbally abuse her. Also during the last four years her boyfriend had begun to date another woman. All of her friends and coworkers knew about this affair before she did. But even after she found out, she continued to live with him because she did not want to disrupt the lives of her children. "I didn't want to cause them to be worried or concerned so I stayed and put my needs off."

She ultimately moved away from him and since that time she had been diagnosed with breast cancer. She had a lumpectomy, radiation, and chemotherapy. "I know why I have cancer," she told me. "I have it because of my living conditions. I have been disrespected and abused for so long. Now I know I've been angry for a long time, but I never knew how to express it. I just didn't know how to do it."

I prescribed for Janice the remedy staphysagria 12 c, three times a day. I asked her to write down her diet and return in two weeks. Her diet diary revealed that she ate modestly and was not getting nearly the amount of vitamins and minerals necessary for someone who had not been ill, and certainly not for someone who had been exposed to the toxicity of radiation treatment. Her diet consisted primarily of coffee, pancakes, milk, and orange juice for breakfast, tuna or smoked turkey sandwiches or shrimp salad for lunch, and fried fish or steak and a baked potato for dinner. She did not drink enough water and ate few vegetables or fruits. As soon as I looked at her diary, it was easy to see another cause of her cancer.

GENERAL DIETARY SUGGESTIONS

For over two decades the National Cancer Institute has maintained that countries with diets high in animal fat have the highest death rates from breast cancer. Animal fats stimulate the production of estrogen from cholesterol, creating excess estrogen in the body. Excess estrogen over the course of a woman's life is associated with an increased risk of breast cancer.

At the same time, various studies have shown that eating larger amounts of fruits and vegetables and adopting a vegetarian diet reduces the risk of most cancers. Vegetarian diets are high in plant estrogen, which decreases the body's own production of estrogen. Fiber is another primary constituent of the vegetarian diet. It binds in the colon to estrogen metabolites, which otherwise would be converted to carcinogens. These carcinogens are reabsorbed into the circulation, increasing the risk of cancer. Another reason why fruits and vegetables are important in the prevention and treatment of cancer is their high vitamin and mineral content. Many fruits and vegetables have indole-3 carbonol, a chemical that changes the way estrogen is metabolized; they also contain high amounts of vitamin C, E, selenium, fiber, and flavonoids that neutralize free radicals.

Foods that I specifically recommend for preventing and treating cancer include brassica family foods (broccoli, cabbage, cauliflower, brussels sprouts, collards, and kale) or cruciferous carotenes (flavonoids) such as orange- and yellow-pigmented fruits and vegetables. These pigmented foods not only stimulate enzymes that destroy carcinogens; they also function as antioxidants and convert to vitamin A in the body. I recommend juicing these vegetables along with beets, celery, dandelion leaves, and sea vegetables. You may also steam or lightly sautee them, but do not boil them!

Soy products are also strongly linked with a lower incidence of cancer, as evidenced by the cancer rates of women from the Far East compared to Western women. Soy products contain compounds that are converted to plant estrogen, which binds to estrogen receptors on the cells and blocks the harmful effects of estrogen. Soybeans also contain a substance called genistein, which interferes with the formation of blood vessels. It is thought that this restriction of blood supply helps inhibit the growth of the tumor.

It is interesting, however, to note the distinctions between Asian men and Western men. While Japanese and Western men have the same incidence of prostate cancer, Japanese men enjoy a significantly lower mortality rate. The difference is due in great part to the consumption of soy products and the adherence to a macrobiotic diet. Macrobiotic diets were popular in the late sixties and seventies and are enjoying a resurgence in this country in our increasingly health-conscious culture. The diet includes soy products but also foods like brown rice, vegetables, and seaweed. But the diet does not promote the consumption of fruits and can be deficient in calcium and vitamin D. So if you adopt a macrobiotic diet, be sure to include a good multivitamin and mineral supplement to make up for these deficiencies, and consult a specialist in this field.

Like soy, lactobacillus acidophilus aids in the prevention and treatment of cancer, particularly of the colon. Acidophilus helps metabolize estrogen in the bowel, helps inhibit toxic bacteria in the colon, and decreases the production of toxic bile acid. If you are not eating a high-fiber diet, which will eliminate the carcinogenic bile acids in the bowel, acidophilus is extremely important to include in your diet.

As stated in previous chapters, you should always follow the diet for your blood type, especially if you are type A or AB. If you are blood type B or O, eliminate red meat and dairy products. Eat primarily fish, beans, vegetables, and fruits. Once every six weeks, go on a detox diet in order to cleanse your system. Now that we have a much better sense of the link between cancer and pesticides, eating organic foods is a critical part of the prevention and treatment of cancer. It is also important to eliminate poisons such as alcohol and refined sugar, since both of these items have been associated with cancer.

Herbal Treatments
and Nutritional Supplements

Shiitake (*Lentinus edodes*) and maitake (*Grifola frondosa*) mushrooms are also found often in the Asian diet. These mushrooms have anticancer activity and are believed to be the reason why there is a lower incidence of cancer particularly in Japan, where research has been definitive on animals with cancerous tumors. The mushrooms activate parts of the immune system that stop cancer cell growth and prevent a recurrence and metastasis of cancer. Specifically, maitake mushrooms seem to be more effective against breast, lung, and liver cancers. Shiitake mushrooms have been shown to prolong the life of patients with recurrent breast, stomach, and colorectal cancer.

Herbs that may be used in combination with conventional treatments include *Allium sativa* (garlic), *Astragalus membranaceus* (astragalus), *Camellia sinensis* (green tea), *Silybum marianum* (milk thistle), and *Curcuma longa* (curcumin or turmeric).

In addition to helping other conditions previously mentioned in this book, garlic has been shown to have antitumor effects. Breast, skin, and colon cancer seem to be most affected by the chemical constituents in garlic.

Astragalus, an herb from China, is used to stimulate the immune system. It has been shown to stimulate the activity of the T-killer cells. In combination with *Panax ginseng* (Korean ginseng), it helps to inhibit the growth of tumors induced by certain carcinogens, by increasing killer cell activity, and maintains the immune cell activity during chemotherapy and radiation treatments. Other herbs that I alternate with ginseng are echinacea and phytolacca.

Green tea is associated with a reduced risk of skin, esophageal, and stomach cancers. One of the ingredients in green tea stimulates the enzymes that absorb free radicals.

The herb milk thistle has been used for decades to assist the nursing mother with milk production. However, it also helps reduce liver damage while promoting protein synthesis. It is a potent antioxidant and protects liver cells and the body against the side effects of conventional treatments.

Curcumin has been shown to be effective in every stage of cancer, from its inception through progression. In some cases it may even promote cancer regression owing to its anticancer effects on various carcinogens and antioxidant qualities. Turmeric reduces the toxicity in cancer patients by helping release harmful agents through one's urine.

All of the above herbs are used in the treatment of all cancers, including lung and prostate cancer. Other herbs specific for the prostate include *Pygeum Africanum* (pygeum), *Serenoa repens* (saw palmetto), and *Foeniculum vulgare* (fennel). Because it is believed that prostate cancer may come from too much male hormone (testosterone), fennel is used in a tincture combined with saw palmetto and pygeum to reduce testosterone. Pygeum is an evergreen tree indigenous to Africa. It is especially useful in BPH to reduce symptoms of frequent nighttime urination or simply difficult or incomplete urination. Pygeum also helps eliminate the accumulation of cholesterol and testosterone, and inflammation in the cancerous or hyperplastic prostate gland. Saw palmetto is native to the West Indies and North America from South Carolina to Florida. Essentially this herb treats the same symptoms as pygeum, and also stops the conversion of testosterone to a more potent and detrimental compound which causes the cells to multiply excessively. Red clover, a phytoestrogen, is also added to this preparation and prescribed at 1–2 teaspoons, three times a day.

Nutrients for the prevention and treatment of cancer include vitamin C and flavonoids, antioxidants (especially vitamins A and E, beta carotene, selenium, zinc, glutathione, or N-acetylcysteine, coenzyme Q10), and omega-3 fatty acids. N-acetylcysteine is converted to glutathione inside your cells. Glutathione is a very powerful antioxidant enzyme that guards against free radicals and toxic buildup in the body. N-acetylcystein protects DNA and supports the liver. It assists cancer patients going through chemotherapy as it protects the healthy cells against the toxic effect of the drugs.

Coenzyme Q10 enables cells to get energy from food. It is also an antioxidant and protects the heart against one of the chemotherapy drugs, Adriamycin. It has been shown to reduce tumor growth, especially in the breast, and is considered a major component in the prevention and treatment of cancer. While I suggest 50 mg, three times a day, for cancer patients, coenzyme Q10 can be found in natural amounts in salmon, mackerel, and sardines.

EXERCISE

Participating in regular exercise conducive to your blood type is an essential part of your healing. It is the regularity that is significant. My patients get a sense of taking charge when they set aside time just for themselves. Exercise helps you pay attention to your body and yourself, not to mention the feelings of vitality that you have after exercise. It also helps you reduce and cope with stress and stimulates the immune system. Unless your cancer has spread to the bone or you have some other condition that contraindicates exercise, do not forget about this valuable part of your cancer treatment.

A FINAL WORD ABOUT CANCER

As with HIV/AIDS, the use of therapy or some support group is essential for treating cancer. As I said earlier, most cancer patients I have seen have been victims of some emotional or physical abuse. And even if they have not been victims of abuse, there is for some reason a tremendous feeling of powerlessness. Their self-concept is poorly developed and confidence is severely lacking. Anger is an uncomfortable feeling for them. While they are afraid to express hatred or feelings of ill will toward another, these same feelings are often directed toward themselves. Or someone in their lives is the target for such harmful, unexpressed emotions. But the feeling of fear and a sense of abandonment are common.

Susceptibility to all of the illnesses mentioned in this book is found in the mental/emotional state of the person, and that state needs to be explored through disciplines that can respond to the need, such as homeopathy and therapy. Sooner or later patients like Paula and Janice realize that somehow they are responsible for their health. This is a step toward healing because it provides a degree of empowerment. Some-how, they understand that they created, promoted, or allowed it to take place, whether by staying in an unhealthy situation too long, or holding on to the hurt and anger after it was over rather than seeking assistance, forgiveness, or letting go. This means they can also create something different, like a better quality of life.

This is not to say that the patient is to blame for the disease. Quite the contrary, as I mentioned in Chapter 3, "Homeopathy," our beliefs and behavior created by stressful situations help create the susceptibility. We learn those behaviors, whether proactive or reactive, from our parents and people in this world. And they learn from their parents, and so on. As I said before, too few of us have been taught how to love and too many of us have been taught how to hate and fear.

It is up to us then to change our beliefs and behavior. The first step toward that change is to become aware of any negative thought patterns that exist. Your first awareness of your behavior patterns may have come when you were first diagnosed with cancer. How did you respond to the diagnosis? I have seen patients who uncover their negative thought patterns and work with them so that change becomes a reality. They are fighters and want something different for their lives. And I have seen patients who do not do that. The former are still living.

To stand up to the diagnosis of cancer takes great courage and strength. I believe psychological intervention is necessary. It helps with prognosis. In addition to therapy and homeopathy, self-help books and personal growth seminars will also be very useful. The phone numbers for seminars can be found on page 251. The books I would recommend are the same books listed in Chapter Eleven, "HIV/AIDS," plus *Getting Well Again,* by Carl O. Simonton, M.D., Stephanie Matthews-Simon-ton, and James L. Creighton. The Simontons advocate psychological intervention as a necessary part of any cancer treatment. Their book covers issues such as resentment, personality types, and beliefs related to cancer and offers techniques such as guided imagery, relaxation, and forgiveness as part of their treatment plan.

It has been noted that the way a patient responds to the diagnosis of breast cancer is the single most important factor in determining the outcome of treatment. Those who are willing to fight for their lives have the greatest survival rate, followed by those who are in denial.

On a subsequent visit, Janice wept as she told me the following: "I have already lost my hair two times. When I lost my hair, I had no distractions. I had to look at the real me. I started learning to accept myself. I think I had been afraid of change. I haven't been flexible in my life. I stayed in situations for fear of change. The cancer helped me—it has made me flexible. I am learning to live each day and appreciate each day. I can hear and see more than before. I am not rushing as much, and now I'm a better judge of character. I am taking care of *my* needs now. I appreciate myself now. I know now that my worthiness is not attached to what I do. I am worthy because I am a child of God."

Janice is a patient who understands that healing involves a change of attitude and lifestyle. Having a life-threatening illness can be a blessing for some people, depending on how they choose to perceive it. If Janice passed away tomorrow, I would still know that she was healed—healed of the self-denial and self-consciousness that runs rampant in our community. We have yet to find a cure for cancer. But with the right preventive care we can take the right measures to reduce the chances of getting this disease and, for people like Janice who are already diagnosed, it is never too late for the healing process to begin.

EPILOGUE

We have come to the end our journey together, for now. I sincerely hope you have gained insight into your life, your health, and what you might do to change them both, if you so choose. Good health is a choice. Not everyone will make that choice as we have seen with my arthritic patient, in Chapter Eight, "Obesity." Some people build their lives, their daily activities, around their illness. Their families, spouses, partners, and friends respond to them based upon this illness. The patterns are set, and to change the patterns means changing how they all interact with one another. There is no judgment if that is what you choose. It just is.

And while those who choose to change their lives may not heal themselves completely, the quality of their lives will improve dramatically. Healing, like illness, takes time. Be patient and be consistent. Healing, like illness, also takes place on many levels, and I have witnessed healing in persons just before they passed over. They were able to heal the hurt and anger of their mental/emotional bodies, though their physical bodies were worn and fragile.

I do not heal everyone. As a matter of fact, I heal no one. I am but a vehicle through which God heals, with the natural substances given to us by God, such as foods, herbs, and minerals. Use them. Heal through them. Allow God's grace to change your life as it has changed mine. You deserve it. You are worthy of wellness. Grace has already been extended to us. But if you need forgiving, please do that. If you need loving, please ask for that. Any dis-ease is an opportunity to go inside and find the "Kingdom of Heaven," to participate in forgiveness and experience gratitude.

Conventional medicine and the power of the nuclear age have outpaced our hearts. In the midst of all the insecurity and instability of this world, which may be manifested in low self-esteem and depression, increased dysfunctional immune systems, or the development of uncontrollable, genetically mutant cells, there is another path, a path to healing.

God bless us all.

I'd like to close with a favorite poem:

I leave you love,
I leave you hope,
I leave you the challenge of developing confidence in one another,
I leave you a thirst for education,
I leave you respect for the use of power,
I leave you faith,
I leave you racial dignity,
I leave you a desire to live harmoniously with your fellow men,
I leave you, finally, a responsibility to our young people.

—Mary McLeod Bethune

COMMONLY ASKED QUESTIONS

1. Do I have to make all of these dietary changes at one time?

No. Make the changes gradually, but consistently, unless you are an all-or-nothing type of person. Make one change at a time, like eliminating red meat, or white flour, or white rice. Then begin to eliminate other substances that you know are not providing proper nutrition.

2. Does following the detox diet mean I can never have a soda or chocolate or white bread?

No, if you eat these things very occasionally. However, if you do not know how to eat one piece of chocolate, try a substitute like carob for a time and wean yourself of it. Then, if you must have a piece of chocolate, do so, a good piece. I find that once people do the detoxification diet and begin to reduce foods that are refined and processed they have less need for refined sweets and foods made with preservatives.

3. If I am a blood type A and like to eat meat, do I have to become vegetarian?

Yes, ultimately, that is the best advice I can give you. But you do not have to be vegetarian by tomorrow. As with all the changes, do one thing at a time. Start by eliminating red meat over a six-month period. Over the next six months reduce and eliminate chicken. Within eighteen months eliminate fish. If you attend a banquet or you are away and your only option is fish, have some, preferably salmon or halibut. But also have as many vegetables as the kitchen will prepare.

4. My grandmother lived to be eighty-nine and she ate everything. Why can't I?

Your grandmother probably didn't have the subtle, uncertain stress that we have in America today. Not to mention the stress of water and air pollution and processed foods. Her food was probably organic, and she got plenty of exercise. She probably didn't smoke, drink, or take recreational drugs, and prescription drugs were not introduced into her system until later in her life. This is a different time, with different stresses—seen and unseen—and we have to guard against the disease that this time in our civilization fosters.

5. After I do the detoxification diet, what will be my normal diet?

If you are blood type A, the detox diet, with some additional fruits, vegetables, nuts, seeds, etc., is your "normal" diet. If you are type B, O, or AB, just add back animal protein in varying amounts. You should eat organic fruits and vegetables, tofu, nuts, seeds, beans, etc., even though you need to also eat animal protein.

6. How long will I be on this blood type diet?

These diets are indicative of lifestyle changes, not just fads that will be in your life for ten days to a month. Everyone needs a diet of organic whole grains and legumes, some animal protein (depending on blood type) and lots of organic vegetables and fruits in order to create and maintain optimal health.

7. How can I find a naturopathic physician for my relative who lives out of the Washington, D.C., area?

Call or write to the American Association of Naturopathic Physicians, the organization that represents naturopaths who have graduated from accredited colleges and universities.

AANP
601 Valley St. Suite 105
Seattle, WA 98109-4229
Monday–Friday 9:00–5:00 PST
Phone (206) 298-0126; Fax (206) 298-0129

8. How can I find a classical homeopathic physician?

Call or write the Homeopathic Academy of Naturopathic Physicians.

HANP
12132 SE Foster Place
Portland, OR 97266

Monday–Friday 9:00–5:00 PST
Phone (503) 761-3298; Fax (503) 762-1929

or

International Foundation for Homeopathy
P.O. Box 7
Edmonds, WA 98020
Monday–Friday 9:00–5:00 PST
Phone (206) 776-4147; Fax (206) 776-1499

or

National Center for Homeopathy
801 North Fairfax Street, Suite 306
Alexandria, VA 22314
Monday–Friday 9:00–4:00 EST
Phone (703) 548-7790; Fax (703) 548-7792

or

American Association for Naturopathic Physicians
601 Valley Street #105
Seattle, WA 90109
Monday–Friday 9:00–5:00 PST
Phone (206) 298-0126
http://www.Naturopathic.org.com

Personal Growth Seminars

Insight Educational Seminars
1-818-735-4966

Temenos Associates
1-703-241-0261

Forum Associates
1-202-833-8000

GLOSSARY

Acetylcysteine (N-Acetylcysteine)   A substance that helps increase the synthesis of glutathione, a powerful antioxidant and liver detoxifier.

Aldosterone   A hormone secreted by the adrenal glands to increase water and salt retention by the kidneys.

Allopathy   A system of medicine that treats the disease with chemical substances (synthetic drugs) producing effects different (and usually opposite) from those of the disease being treated; e.g., *anti*biotics, *anti*histamine.

Allopathic, conventional, orthodox physician   A person who practices allopathic medicine.

Amino acids   Organic compounds occurring naturally in plant and animal tissues, and forming the main component of protein.

Angiotensin   A polypeptide (amino acid) that aids in the regulation of blood pressure and stimulates the secretion of aldosterone by the adrenal cortex, causing the kidneys to retain salt and water and therefore increasing arterial pressure.

Anthocyanidins   Antioxidant flavinoids ("plant pigment" is a general term for these compounds) responsible for the varying colors of fruits like blackberries, blueberries, and cherries, and of vegetables like red and yellow peppers and sweet potatoes.

Antibodies   Chemicals called immunoglobulins, made by the cells of the immune system to identify and eliminate foreign substances in the body. People are classified into blood groups O, B, and A, and AB, according to the antibodies we create to destroy other red blood cells that are foreign to our bodies. For example, blood from a person who is Group A would cause the blood of a person with Group B blood to clump, and vice-versa.

Antigen   Any substance (i.e., bacteria, foreign proteins, toxins) that stimulates the immune system to form antibodies when it is introduced into the body.

Antimony   A chemical element forming different medicinal and poisonous salts that, when ingested, can create symptoms of arsenic poisoning; antimony was used by allopathic physicians as an agent to induce vomiting in the 1700s and 1800s.

Antioxidants   Substances (vitamins, minerals, and enzymes) that protect the body from the damage of free radicals (atoms or groups of atoms that can cause damage to our cells; formed by exposure to radiation and toxic chemicals, as well as by overexposure to the sun).

Arachidonic acid   An essential fatty acid, found only in land animal fat, that the body uses to produce pro-inflammatory series-2 prostaglandins.

AZT   A drug, zidovudine, used to treat HIV-infected people, specifically to increase the T4 cells by interfering with the reproduction of HIV. The brand name is Retrovir.

Bloodletting   The act of letting blood by opening a vein, referring to the use of leeches in the 1700s and 1800s; used in conjunction with substances like antimony and mercury for purging.

Chiropractic medicine   A system of medicine that attributes disease to the dysfunction of the nervous system and uses manipulation of the vertebral column and other body structures to restore health.

Complementary medicine   Systems of medicine including naturopathy, homeopathy, Oriental and Western herbal medicine, and chiropractic medicine.

Decoction   A preparation made by boiling, i.e., adding an herb to boiling water as in a tea.

Dysmenorrhea   Painful menstruation (menses).

Eclectic medicine   A system of medicine that was founded upon the work of Samuel Thomson, who believed in the use of herbs to restore the body's energy.

Eicosapentaenoic acid (EPA)   An essential fatty acid that is necessary to make the series-3 prostaglandins; it is made from linolenic acid.

Essential fatty acids   Fatty acids that are necessary for the production of prostaglandins but are not made by the body.

Glutathione (L-Glutathione)   An antioxidant that inhibits the formation of free radicals that come from cigarette smoking or radiation.

Homeopathy   A system of medicine that uses minute doses of natural substances (herbs, minerals, or animal secretions) which are capable of producing in healthy persons the same symptoms (mental, emotional, and physical) of the disease of the person being treated.

Homeostasis   The maintenance of stability or balance, especially in the physiological system of humans because of the coordinated responses of its organs in the face of a situation or stimuli that is capable of disturbing normal functioning.

Hydrotherapy   The use of water in any form or temperature for the treatment of disease, internally (colonic irrigation) or externally (bath or shower).

Hyperplasia   Abnormal increase in the number of normal cells in an organ or tissue.

Hypertrophy   Enlargement of an organ or part due to increase in the size of its cells.

Ischemia   Deficiency of blood to a part due to constriction or obstruction of a blood vessel.

Leukotrienes   Chemical mediators produced by the white blood cells in an immune response to antigens, causing inflammatory reactions, allergic asthma, and other reactions.

Metastasis   The movement of disease from one organ or part of the body to another part not directly connected, due to the transfer of the microorganism or the transfer of cells, as in the case of cancer.

Naturopathy   A system of medicine that believes in the body's innate intelligence to heal itself using natural substances such as herbs, foods, water, exercise, manipulation, and homeopathy; naturopathy does not employ synthetic drugs or surgery.

Pectin   A fiber found in fruits that increases the secretion of digestive enzymes and decreases transmit time of the bowel, thus decreasing the opportunity for toxic compounds to be absorbed into the blood.

Placebo   An inactive substance given to a patient to satisfy the patient's psychological need for drug therapy; also used in control studies to determine the efficacy of medicinal substances being tested.

Prostaglandins   A group of unsaturated fatty acids found in the body that control inflammatory responses and body temperature, as well as other physiological functions.

Purines   Constituents of nucleoproteins (single proteins combined with nucleic acid). Uric acid is the final breakdown of purine metabolism.

Renin   An enzyme that assists in the production of angiotensin and therefore helps to regulate blood pressure. The **renin-angiotensin system** is activated when there is a decrease in arterial pressure or a decrease in the quantity of sodium in the body fluids. The kidneys secrete renin, which acts on a plasma protein and forms angiotensin; this constricts blood vessels and causes the kidneys to retain salt and water.

Reverse transcriptase   One of the enzymes inside the viral core (where the genetic code is located) of the HIV; changes the genetic code of the virus into that of the human host cell.

Solanaceae plants   Also referred to as the deadly nightshade family of plants. Includes tomatoes, potatoes, eggplant, peppers, and tobacco. Can aggravate arthritic conditions.

Sympathetic nervous system   A part of the autonomic nervous system that regulates circulation and volume of blood flow through tissues of the body. Plays a major role in cardiovascular function.

Vitalism   A philosophy at the core of naturopathy and homeopathy, holding that life is more than a series of biochemical reactions; but rather life, and all of the reactions that sustain life, is coordinated and organized by a force or spirit.

Recipes

Cooking Times and Proportions for Grains and Legumes

GRAIN (1 CUP DRY MEASURE)	WATER (CUPS)	COOKING TIME (SOAK BEANS OVERNIGHT)
Barley	3	1 hr. 15 min.
Black Beans	4	1½ hr.
Brown Rice	2	45 min.
Bulgur	2	15 min.
Chickpeas	4	3 hr.
Cornmeal	2½–3	25 min.
Cracked Wheat	2	25 min.
Kasha/Buckwheat	2	15 min.
Kidney Beans	3	1½ hr.
Lentils and Split Peas	3	1 hr.
Lima Beans	2	¾ hr.
Millet	2½	25 min.
Oatmeal	1	20 min.
Pinto Beans	3	2 hr.
Soya Beans	4	3 hr. or more
Soy Grits	2	15 min.
White Navy Beans	3	1½ hr.
Wild Rice	3	1 hr.

Turn a bean pot into a stew by adding chopped vegetables/herbs for the last half hour.

MILLET AND BUCKWHEAT BREAKFAST

½ cup millet
½ cup buckwheat
½ teaspoon sea salt
Flax seeds (optional)
1 cup diced sweet vegetables, sautéed in ghee
4 cups water

Wash grains well and dry-roast if desired for more flavor. Place grains, sea salt, and flax seeds in a medium-size saucepan, cover with water, and soak overnight. You can also sauté vegetables but wait till morning to add. Next morning, drain grains and add vegetables and 4 cups water to the pan. Place over low heat, uncovered, and simmer 30 minutes. This recipe can be cooking while you are getting dressed.

&

SOYBEAN WAFFLES

2¼ cups water
1 cup soybeans (soaked overnight)
1½ cups rolled oats, uncooked
1 tablespoon oil
½ teaspoon salt

Blend all ingredients for ½ minute. Let sit 5–10 minutes in well-greased waffle iron, cook each waffle 8 minutes until golden brown.

&

BRAN MUFFINS

1 cup whole wheat flour
1 teaspoon baking soda
1½ cups bran
½ cup raisins
1 egg, well beaten

½ cup molasses or honey
¾ cup milk
2 tablespoons butter

Preheat the oven to 400°F. Mix together dry ingredients and raisins and moisten with egg and molasses (or honey), milk, and butter. Stir only enough to blend. Bake in well-greased muffin tins for 20–30 minutes until golden brown.

BREAKFAST VARIATIONS

- ⚬ Cooked oatmeal, plain
- ⚬ Cooked millet with a sprinkle of wheat germ and wheat bran
- ⚬ Oatmeal cooked in soybean milk, with a sprinkle of sunflower seeds
- ⚬ Poached or hard-boiled egg; serve with celery, cucumber, carrot, or zucchini strips with a bit of tofu dressing
- ⚬ Cooked oatmeal, with crumbled tofu and sunflower seeds

APPETIZERS

GUACAMOLE DELIGHT

1 large fresh tomato, skinned and finely chopped
4 green onions, finely chopped
Juice of ½ lemon
1 teaspoon tamari
3 dashes of Tabasco sauce
¼ teaspoon pepper
Salt to taste (consider sea salt)
Dash of cayenne
3 ripe avocados, skinned, pitted, and mashed (save the pits)

Mix the tomato and onions together in a bowl. Add the next six ingredients. Mix together.

Add the avocado and mix well.

NOTE: To prevent discoloration, add the avocado pits. Remove the pits just before serving. A great vegetable or chip dip.

ENTREES

VEGGIE BURGER

½ cup soaked garbanzo beans*
½ cup water
1 cup rolled oats, uncooked
1 cup finely chopped walnuts
1 medium onion, minced
4 tablespoons rice milk
1 teaspoon dried sage
1 tablespoon soy sauce
Salt and pepper to taste

Whiz the first two ingredients in a blender. Remove to a bowl. Add remaining ingredients and mix with a spoon. Use ice cream scoop to form patties. Brown on both sides over medium heat. Serve on burger buns with all the trimmings or in a casserole with gravy over the top, baking 30 minutes at 350°F.

NOTE: 7.2 grams of protein and 226 calories per patty.

MILLET WITH SWEET VEGETABLES

2 cups millet (washed well and drained well)
2 medium onions, finely chopped
1 small butternut squash, skinned, seeded, and diced
3 carrots, diced
1½ teaspoons sea salt
5½ cups water
1–2 tablespoons ghee or butter

*¼ cup dry garbanzo beans soaked 8 hours in water will yield ½ cup drained beans.

Dry-roast millet in skillet if desired to increase flavor. Into pressure cooker, layer onions, squash, carrots, and millet. Dissolve sea salt in water and gently pour water around sides of millet and vegetables. Close cover and bring pressure cooker up to pressure. Cook over low heat for 30 minutes. Remove, let pressure drop and open lid. Fold in ghee or butter. Stir well, then serve.

NOTE: This dish can also be prepared in a saucepan. Increase the amount of water to 6 cups and follow the same directions.

OPTION: Consistency is even creamier if you puree millet/veggie mixture with ghee in a blender.

VARIATION: Add a strip of Kombu sea vegetable. It will not be quite as sweet but it is even healthier.

IMPORTANT: This dish nourishes the spleen/pancreas and stomach. It is the most healing way to cook millet. With candida, millet is most easily tolerated when the sweet vegetables (onions, carrots, and butternut squash) are added.

STUFFED TROUT

Take whole fresh trout and stuff with a julienne of celery, carrots, and slivered mushrooms. To season, add chopped dill, parsley, and minced garlic, plus a generous squeeze of lemon. Bake until flaky and top with some seasame seeds and more lemon.

SESAME TOFU

2 pounds firm tofu, cubed
⅓ cup tamari
¼ cup olive oil
2 cloves garlic, minced
1 tablespoon grated gingerroot
1 cup grand sesame seeds

Marinate the tofu for 2 hours in a mixture of tamari, olive oil, garlic, and gingerroot. Drain the marinade from the tofu. Roll the cubes in the sesame seeds.

Preheat the oven to 350°F. Bake the tofu on an oiled cookie sheet for 15 minutes.

◦ᴥ

MISO POACHED CHICKEN

Take a chicken breast, and debone it. In a frying pan pour in a little water, and dissolve some miso. Add some minced garlic, sesame seeds, lemon, basil, and mushrooms. Bring the broth to a boil and add the deboned chicken; cover and simmer until tender. Remove chicken to a plate, and ladle a few tablespoons of broth over it. Garnish with the poached mushrooms, some sesame seeds, and a sprinkle of chopped fresh parsley.

◦ᴥ

ROMAINE LEAVES STUFFED WITH FISH AND VEGETABLES

Steam large romaine leaves until wilted. Mince parsley, celery, mushrooms, garlic, and dill to taste, season with lemon juice. Take a piece of fish (a fillet), and put some of the vegetable mixture on the fish. Place the fillet on a romaine leaf, roll up, and secure with a toothpick. Bake until flaky. The fish may then be sprinkled with slivered almonds and a squeeze of lemon juice.

◦ᴥ

CREAMY TAHINI RICE

1 medium onion, chopped
1 cup mixed nuts (almonds, seeds)
3 cups cooked rice

2 tablespoons tamari
⅓ cup tahini
⅓ cup water

Mix together all the ingredients. Cook gently in saucepan until it is heated through and the sauce is thick and creamy around the grain.

NOTE: This recipe may also be served with beans.

SPAGHETTI SQUASH CASSEROLE

1 medium-sized spaghetti squash
4–6 cups your favorite tomato sauce, made with onions, garlic, and herbs
Grated/Cheddar or Parmesan cheese

Preheat the oven to 350°F. Bake the squash, whole, about 1½ hours or until tender. When cooked, cut open, remove seedy center, and scoop out pulp.

Pour the tomato sauce over the squash and top with grated Cheddar or Parmesan cheese. Return to the 350° oven until cheese browns.

VARIATION: Add carrots and celery to your tomato sauce or try extra-firm tofu crumbled or cut into small pieces.

BAKED NUT MEAT

1 egg
1 cup Thick Sauce (see recipe)
½ pound ground cashews
6 ounces ground nuts (your choice)
4 ounces bread crumbs
½ cup sliced mushrooms
1 cup sliced sautéed scallions
½ cup minced fresh parsley

2 teaspoons chopped kelp
2 teaspoons chopped basil
2 teaspoons chopped chervil
Dash of pepper
Sesame seeds
Grated cheese

Preheat the oven to 350°F. In a large bowl, beat the egg, and mix with all the other ingredients except the sesame seeds and grated cheese. Turn the mixture into a well-greased 9-inch pie dish. Sprinkle with lots of sesame seeds and grated cheese. Bake for 50 minutes.

❧

EGGPLANT CASSEROLE

1 large eggplant, cut into small chunks
2–3 cups stewed tomatoes
6 mushrooms, sliced
1 onion, chopped
Salt and pepper to taste
1 cup grated Romano cheese (or Cheddar if you prefer)

In a medium size saucepan, simmer eggplant and tomatoes over low heat until eggplant is soft and clear-looking, about 15 minutes. Meanwhile saute mushrooms and onion in olive oil in a small skillet until tender. Preheat the oven to 350°F. Pour the eggplant and tomatoes, the mushroom and onion mixture, and the seasonings into a greased casserole dish. Top with grated cheese and bake for 20 minutes.

ENTREE VARIATIONS

- ❧ Spinach salad with mushrooms, mung bean sprouts, and sunflower seeds, with cheese cubes or egg slices, and crumbled tofu
  Lemon and oil dressing
- ❧ Tofu burger
  Slice of bread
  Salad

❧ Chickpea dip served with vegetables: carrots, celery, zuc-
chini, cucumbers, broccoli, or mushrooms
Flat bread crackers
❧ Steamed vegetables and tofu with sunflower seeds
Baked potato or brown rice
❧ Salad and tofu cubes
Vegetarian soup with lentils or pinto beans
❧ Salad with sliced egg and sunflower seeds and almonds
Tofu dressing
❧ Salad with tofu cubes with cold brown rice and slivered al-
monds
Tofu dressing or lemon and oil dressing
❧ Salad with cubes of sweet potato and sunflower seeds
Tofu dressing or lemon and oil dressing
❧ Salad with cubes of tofu and garbanzo beans
Slice of bread

Soup

Linda's (Vegetable) Soup

1 onion, chopped
1 green pepper, chopped
2 tablespoons oil
1½ teaspoons chopped basil
1 tablespoon chopped summer savory
8 cups vegetable stock
1 potato, diced
2 stalks celery, chopped
1 carrot, sliced
¼ cup barley
⅓ cup lima beans
¼ cup chopped parsley
Salt and pepper to taste

Saute onion and green pepper in oil for a few minutes. Add basil and
savory. Add to stock along with the rest of the ingredients. Heat to

boiling, then simmer until barley and beans are tender (it might be best to add barley and beans 15 minutes before vegetables).

ACCOMPANIMENTS

CARROTS WITH FENNEL

8–10 carrots
Juice of 1 lemon
1½ tablespoons chopped fresh fennel (or 1 teaspoon dried)
2 tablespoons institute spread

Preheat the oven to 350°F. Slice carrots into julienne strips. Place in a small baking dish, sprinkle with lemon juice and fennel. Dot with institute spread. Cover tightly and bake for 40 minutes or until tender, stirring once or twice during cooking.

∾

BAKED RICE BALLS

1 cup cooked brown rice
1 egg, lightly beaten
½ teaspoon salt
½ cup almonds
½ cup mashed tofu
1 teaspoon lemon juice
½ cup sesame seeds (roasted)

Combine all the ingredients except the sesame seeds and shape into balls. Roll in sesame seeds and bake on an oiled cookie sheet for 30 minutes.

Serve with Tahini Gravy or Almond Gravy (see recipes).

∾

PILAF (BULGUR/MILLET, WHEAT, OR RICE)

Pilaf can be made with any grain. See cooking chart to adjust cooking instructions.

Dice 1 carrot, 1 onion, 1 stalk celery, ¼ cup chopped mushrooms, and 2 green onions. Place in a saucepan 1½ tablespoons oil, vegetables, 1 bay leaf, 1 teaspoon sea salt, and 1¾ cups water or vegetable stock. Bring to a boil, then simmer, covered, for 5 minutes. Add grain (1 cup of raw bulgur/millet, cracked wheat, or rice) and bring to a boil, then cook, covered, over very low heat until ready.

SALADS

KALE GREENS SALAD

2 pounds kale
½ cup chopped scallions
1 large red pepper, cut in large pieces
1 large yellow pepper, cut in large pieces
½ cup tamari
¼ cup olive oil
¼ cup lemon juice
4 large cloves garlic, chopped

Clean the greens in warm water and tear into bite-size pieces. Remove excess water from the greens by blotting them with a paper towel.

Mix the scallions, peppers, and greens together. Put the tamari sauce, olive oil, lemon juice, and garlic in a jar with a tight-fitting lid and shake it until it mixes together. Pour over the vegetables.

Refrigerate for at least 2 hours; overnight is preferable.

Serve chilled.

TOFU-EGG SALAD

1 hard-boiled egg, chopped
½ carrot, diced

½ stalk celery, diced
2 tablespoons chopped parsley
2 tablespoons chopped dill
Creamy Tofu Dressing (see recipe), enough to moisten ingredients
1 green onion, chopped
A few sunflower seeds (optional)
A little tamari (optional)

Combine all the ingredients in a small bowl. Serve on a bed of greens.

BASIC RICE SALAD

2 cups cooked brown rice
3 tablespoons oil
3 tablespoons lemon juice
¼ cup chopped parsley
¼ cup chopped scallions
1 cup each of the following: cooked beans, carrots, raw peas, diced celery,
    diced cooked cauliflower or broccoli
Fresh, chopped garlic (optional)
2 tablespoons tamari (optional)
Herbs to taste (dill, basil, and so on)
Nuts/seeds as garnish (optional)

Mix all the ingredients. Marinate at least 2 hours in the refrigerator. Serve chilled.

CHICKPEA SALAD

¼ cup minced parsley
¼ cup minced onion
1 large garlic clove, minced
6 tablespoons lemon juice
5 tablespoons oil

⅛ teaspoon cayenne
½ teaspoon salt
3 cups drained cooked chickpeas

Combine all the ingredients except the chickpeas and mix well. Add the chickpeas and stir. Adjust seasonings to taste.

KIDNEY, GARBANZO, AND STRING BEAN SALAD

1½ cups cooked kidney beans
1½ cups cooked garbanzo beans
2 cups freshly steamed string beans
½ clove garlic, minced
½ cup oil
1 cup chopped vegetables (parsley, celery, onion, and mushrooms)
½ cup lemon or cider vinegar
1 teaspoon chopped basil
1 teaspoon chopped oregano

Combine all the ingredients. Marinate in the refrigerator overnight. Serve cold.

SAUCES/DRESSINGS

TAHINI SALAD DRESSING

½ cup lemon juice
¼ cup olive oil
2 tablespoons raw sesame butter
2 tablespoons honey
2 tablespoons water
Dash of tamari

Combine the ingredients. Mix well and serve.

THICK SAUCE

2 ounces butter
2 cloves chopped garlic
2 ounces whole wheat flour
½ pint milk

Melt butter with garlic in small pan over low heat. Stir in flour. Keep stirring for 2 minutes then stir in liquid. Cook gently but thoroughly until the paste comes free from the sides of the pan.

⬧

QUICK YOGURT SAUCE

1 cup chilled yogurt
⅓ cup grated Cheddar cheese (or your favorite cheese)
¼ teaspoon chopped thyme
¼ teaspoon chopped sage
¼ teaspoon chopped basil
½ teaspoon chopped dill weed
1–1½ teaspoons tamari

Mix all the ingredients and serve as a topping on vegetables or Veggie Burger (see recipe).

⬧

TAHINI GRAVY

2 teaspoons arrowroot or cornstarch
1½ tablespoons tamari
1 cup water or vegetable stock
2 tablespoons tahini

Make a paste of starch and tamari, gradually stir in liquid and cook over a moderate heat until it thickens. Stir in tahini. Cool 5 minutes and serve.

⬧

ALMOND GRAVY

6 tablespoons finely ground raw almonds
1¼ to 1½ cups water
1 tablespoon arrowroot or cornstarch
2 tablespoons tamari
Salt to taste
Lemon juice to taste

Gradually add 1¼ cups water to finely ground nuts to make a smooth "milk." Mix starch with a little of the almond milk to make a thin paste. Stir in remaining milk and tamari. Cook over low heat gently until thickened. If too thick, add ¼ cup extra water. Season with salt and lemon juice.

CREAMY TOFU DRESSING

8 ounces tofu
3 tablespoons lemon juice or 2 tablespoons cider vinegar plus 1 tablespoon
    lemon juice
¼ teaspoon dry mustard
Pinch of salt
1 tablespoon tamari
¼ cup oil
⅓ cup water

Combine all the ingredients except the oil and water in a food processor or a blender. Puree until smooth, gradually adding oil. Add ⅓ cup water. Dressing should be of a thick pouring consistency. If necessary, add more water.

TOFU MAYONNAISE

¼ cup oil
¼ teaspoon mustard powder

Dash each of cayenne and kelp powder
2 tablespoons lemon juice
1 block well-dried tofu

Blend all the ingredients well. Add herbs or garlic if desired.

BLENDER HERB DRESSING

2 tablespoons lemon juice or cider vinegar
¼ cup chopped watercress
2 tablespoons chopped green onions
1 egg yolk
¼ cup oil
1 teaspoon each chopped savory, parsley, tarragon, dill

Blend all the ingredients in a blender until well mixed.

NATURAL HERB DRESSING

¼ teaspoon each minced anise seed, dill weed, spearmint, tarragon
1⅓ cups oil
⅔ cup lemon juice
1 clove minced garlic (optional)

Crush anise seed and other herbs (including garlic, if desired) into fine pieces and place in jar with a tight-fitting lid. Add oil and lemon juice. Shake well and refrigerate.

DESSERTS

CAROB FUDGE

2 cups peanut butter
½ cup chopped almonds

Honey to taste
Carob to taste (be generous if you want a real rich chocolate-like flavor)

Mix the ingredients well and pat into a small pan. Refrigerate first to firm, cut in squares, and enjoy. If you can't wait that long it's okay—it's still a treat.

VARIATION: Add unsweetened coconut or raisins. Or substitute 1 cup peanut butter and 1 cup sesame or sunflower butter for the 2 cups peanut butter.

~&

Fruit Shake

2 ripe bananas
Chopped nuts

Peel and freeze several super-ripe bananas. Put in blender and add other frozen fruits if you like—also sprinkle in some nuts. Blend until smooth.

~&

Dried Apple-Boiled Cider Pie

Facts you should know:
    Boiled cider is the tangy syrup made by boiling fresh unpasteurized cider in an uncovered pot until it is reduced to approximately one fifth its original volume and is about the consistency of maple syrup. In fact, by continued boiling one can go on to create treats such as cider jelly and cider chew candies. Boiled cider is very good on waffles, in cooking, flavoring, or any other idea you can think up. After boiling it can be sealed in canning jars to preserve or kept in the refrigerator for quite a while. Here's a recipe for a tangy, pungent, rich tart pie that has a tendency to make other apple pies seem insipid by comparison. The maple sugar is optional if you have a low tolerance for sweets, although it adds a good flavor.

NOTE: The dried apples have to be soaked overnight before making the pie.

Whole grain pastry for 2 (9-inch) pie crusts
¼ cup maple sugar (optional)
3 tablespoons cornstarch
½ cup boiled cider
1½ cups boiling water
1 egg, beaten
1 tablespoon melted butter
½ pound organic dried apples, soaked overnight
Cinnamon to taste
Nutmeg to taste
Allspice to taste
Nuts (optional)

Preheat the oven to 425°F. Fit bottom crust into a 9-inch pie pan. Combine the maple sugar and cornstarch in a bowl. Add the boiled cider and water. Mix. Then add the egg and butter. Lay out apples on the crust in the pan and add the filling. Place the top crust on top and crimp edges tightly. Slash cuts in the top crust and bake for 40 minutes or until done.

OTHER RECIPES

EGGLESS CORN BREAD

½ teaspoon salt
1 tablespoon soy flour
1 tablespoon baking powder
2 cups whole wheat pastry flour
3 cups cornmeal
¾ cup honey
¼ pound butter or margarine
3 cups soy milk

Preheat the oven to 350°F. Mix the dry ingredients. Add honey, butter, and milk in that order to dry ingredients. Pour into a well-greased 10 × 12-inch pan. Bake for 40 minutes or until firm to touch.

TOFU SPREAD

8 ounces tofu, pressed and mashed
Juice of ½ lemon or lime, or more to taste
1 garlic clove, minced
3 tablespoons minced parsley
3 tablespoons minced dill
⅓ cup chopped celery
1 teaspoon any dried herb
A few drops of cold-pressed olive oil
1 teaspoon tamari (optional)
¼ cup sesame seeds (optional)
½ cup alfalfa sprouts

Combine all the ingredients in a bowl. Chill for a few hours for improved flavor. Delicious on rice cakes, in a sandwich, or in a salad.

STEAM/FRY METHOD FOR WOK COOKING

Pour ½ cup water in wok. Add some miso to flavor. Add 1 tablespoon oil. Over low heat, add vegetables in order of cooking times; tofu, fish, or chicken may be added. Garlic and herbs may also be added. A little tahini is nice too. Sesame, sunflower, or slivered almonds may be added near end of cooking time.

BIBLIOGRAPHY

INTRODUCTION

Angelou, Maya. *Wouldn't Take Nothin' for My Journey Now.* New York: Random House, 1993.

Bennett, Nicholas, and Roger J. Neale. "The Effects of Food upon Behavior Nutrition and Crime." *Health,* 10:1994, pp. 49–86.

Higginbotham, A. Leon, Jr. *In the Matter of Color, Race and the American Legal Process: The Colonial Period.* New York: Oxford University Press, 1978.

Robinson, J., and A. Ferguson. "Food Sensitivity and the Nervous System: Hyperactivity, Addiction and Criminal Behavior." *Nutrition Research Reviews* V, 203–23, 1992.

Schauss, A. *Diet, Crime and Delinquency.* Washington: Life Sciences Press, 1981.

CHAPTER ONE
WHAT IS HEALTH? A NATUROPATHIC PERSPECTIVE

Pizzorno, Joseph E., N.D., and Michael T. Murray, N.D. *A Textbook of Natural Medicine.* Seattle: John Bastyr Publications, 1987.

Roger, John, and Peter McWilliams. *Wealth 101.* Los Angeles: Prelude Press, 1992.

CHAPTER TWO
NATUROPATHY: THE ROOTS

Blassingame, John W., ed. *Slave Testimony: Two Centuries of Letters, Speeches, Interviews and Autobiographies.* Baton Rouge, La.: Louisiana State University Press, 1977.

Boyd, Eddie L., Leslie L. Shimp, and Marvie Jarmon Hackney. *Home Remedies and the Black Elderly: A Reference Manual for Health Care Providers.* Institute of Gerontology and College of Pharmacy. Ann Arbor: University of Michigan Press, 1985.

Fontenot, Wonda L. *Secret Doctors: Ethnomedicine of African Americans.* Westport, Conn.: Bergin and Garvey, 1944.

Genovese, Elizabeth Fox. *Within the Plantation Household: Black and White Women of the Old South.* Chapel Hill, N.C.: University of North Carolina Press, 1988.

Genovese, Eugene D. *Roll Jordon Roll: The World the Slaves Made.* New York: Vintage Books, 1974.

Gillespie, Charles C., ed. *Dictionary of Scientific Biography.* Vol. XI. Princeton, N.J.: Scribner Press, 1975.

Grieve, M. *A Modern Herbal.* Vols. I and II. New York: Dover Publications, 1971.

Jordan, Weymouth T. "Plantation Medicine in the Old South." *The Alabama Review,* Vol. III, no. 2, 1950.

King, William Harvey, M.D., LL.D. *History of Homeopathy and Its Institutions in America.* New York: Lewis Publishing Company, 1905.

Knuts-Cheraux, A. W., B.S., M.D., N.D., ed. *Naturae Medicina and Naturopathic Dispensatory.* Yellow Springs, Ohio: Antioch Press, 1953.

"Negro Caezar's Cure for the Bite of a Rattlesnake." In *People's Advocate,* October 25, 1879, p. 1.

Numbers, R., and D. Amundsen, eds. *Caring and Curing: Health and Medicine in the Western Religious Traditions.* New York: Macmillan, 1986.

Payne-Jackson, Arvilla, and John Lee. *Folk Wisdom and Mother Wit.* Westport, Conn.: Greenwood Press, 1993.

Pizzorno, Joseph E., N.D., and Michael T. Murray, N.D. *A Textbook of Natural Medicine.* Seattle: John Bastyr Publications, 1987.

Postell, William. *The Health of Slaves on Southern Plantations.* Baton Rouge, La.: Louisiana State University Press, 1951.

Primm, Beny J. "Poverty, Folk Remedies and Drug Misuse Among the Black Elderly." In *Health and the Black Aged,* Wilbur H. Watson, John Skinner, Irene Lewis, and Shirley A. Wesley, eds. Pp. 63–70. Washington, D.C.: DC National Center on Black Aged, 1977.

Rawick, George P., ed. *The American Slave.* Westport, Conn.: Greenwood Press, 1972.

Robinson, Jean. "Black Healers During the Colonial Period & Early 19th Century America," Ph.D. Dissertation, Southern Illinois University, 1979.

Savitt, Todd L. *Medicine and Slavery: The Diseases and Health Care of Blacks in Antebellum Virginia.* Urbana, Ill.: University of Illinois Press, 1978.

Snow, Loudell F. *Walkin' over Medicine.* Boulder, Colo.: Westview Press, 1993.

Swados, Felice. "Negro Health on the Ante-Bellum Plantations." *Bulletin of the History of Medicine,* 10:1941. Baltimore, Md.: Johns Hopkins University Press, pp. 460–72.

Swaim, William. *A Treatise on the Alternative and Curative Virtues of Swaim's Panacea and Its Application to the Different Diseases of the Human System.* Philadelphia: 1842.

Terrell, Suzanne J. *This Other Kind of Doctor: Traditional Medical Systems in Black Neighborhoods in Austin, Texas.* New York: AMS Press, 1990.

Thacker, Emily. *Home Remedies from the Old South.* Canton, Ohio: Tresco Publishers, 1993.

Villarosa, Linda, ed. *Body & Soul: The Black Women's Guide to Physical Health & Emotional Well-Being.* New York: Harper Perennial, 1994.

Walker, Margaret. *Jubilee.* Boston: Houghton Mifflin, 1966.

Watson, Wilbur H. "Aging and Race." *Social Action,* 30, 4 (1971), pp. 20–30.

———, ed. *Black Folk Medicine: The Therapeutic Significance of Faith and Trust.* New Brunswick, N.J.: Transaction Books, 1984.

Wesley, John. *Primitive Physic.* Philadelphia: Parry Hall, 1793, reprint 1958.

Westmacott, Richard. *African American Gardens and Yards in the Rural South.* Knoxville, Tenn.: University of Tennessee Press, 1992.

White, Evelyn C., ed. *Black Women's Health Book: Speaking for Ourselves.* Seattle: Seal Press, 1990.

Williams, Brett, ed. *The Politics of Culture.* Washington, D.C.: Smithsonian Institution Press, 1991.

CHAPTER THREE
HOMEOPATHY

Allen T. F., M.D. *The Encyclopedia of Pure Materia Medica.* New Delhi, India: B. Jain Publishing, 1992.

Bellavite, Paola, M.D. "Homeopathy: A Frontier in Medical Science, Chapter 3—Is Homeopathy Effective?" *Townsend Letter: for Doctors and Patients,* 160: Nov. 1996, p. 56.

Davenas, E., F. Beauvais, J. Amara, M. Oberbaum, B. Robinzon, A. Miadonna, A. Tedeschi, B. Pomeranz, P. Fortner, P. Belon, J. Sainte-Laudy, B. Poltevin, and J. Benveniste. "Human Basophil Degranulation Triggered by Very Dilute Antiserum Against IgE." *Nature,* vol. 333(6176): 1988, pp. 816–18.

Hahnemann, Samuel. *Organon of Medicine,* 6th ed. Jost Kunzli, M.D., Alain Naude, and Peter Pendleton, eds. Boston: Houghton-Mifflin, 1982.

———. *The Lesser Writings of Samuel Hahnemann.* New York: William Radde, 1852.

Kent, James Tyler, A.M., M.D. *New Remedies, Clinical Cases, Lesser Writings, Aphorisms and Precepts.* Chicago: Ehrhardt and Karl, 1926.

King, William Harvey, M.D., LL.D. *History of Homeopathy and Its Institutions in America,* 4 vols. New York: Lewis Publishing Company, 1905.

Matthews, Robert. "Doctor Defies Doubters on Homeopathy." *Sunday London Telegraph,* News section, July 3, 1994, p. 12.

Morrison, Roger. *Desktop Guide to Keynotes and Confirmatory Symptoms.* Albany, Calif.: Hahnemann Clinic Publishing, 1993.

Starr, Paul. *The Social Transformation of American Medicine.* New York: Basic Books, 1982.

Vithoulkas, George. *The Science of Homeopathy.* New York: Grove Press, 1980.

CHAPTER FOUR
NUTRITION AND YOUR BLOOD TYPE

D'Adamo, James, M.D. *The D'Adamo Diet.* Toronto: McGraw-Hill Ryerson, 1989.

———. *One Man's Food . . . Is Someone Else's Poison.* Toronto: Health Thru Herbs, 1980.

D'Adamo, Peter J., M.D. *Eat Right 4 Your Type.* New York: Putnam, 1996.

Dufty, William. *Sugar Blues.* New York: Warner Books, 1975.

Matsen, John, N.D. *Eating Alive.* Vancouver: Compton Books, 1987.

CHAPTER FIVE

STRESS

Clinton, William Jefferson, in "Rift Between Blacks, Whites 'Is Tearing at the Heart of America.'" *Washington Post,* October 17, 1995, Section A, p. 13.

Davis, George, and Glegg Watson. *Black Life in Corporate America: Swimming in the Mainstream.* Prescott, Ariz.: Anchor Books, 1982.

Declining Economic Status of Black Children: Examining the Change. Washington, D.C.: Joint Center for Political and Economic Studies, 1990.

Hertzberg, Hendrik, and Henry Louis Gates, Jr. "The African American Century." *The New Yorker,* April 29 and May 6, 1996, pp. 9–10.

Higginbotham, A. Leon, Jr. "Why I Didn't March." *Washington Post,* October 17, 1995, Section A, p. 13.

Hornor, Louise L. *Black Americans: A Statistical Sourcebook.* Washington, D.C.: Information Publications, 1994, pp. 56, 57, 258–73.

Klonoff, Elizabeth A., and Hope Landrine. "The Schedule of Racist Events: A Measure of Racial Discrimination and a Study of Its Negative Physical and Mental Health Consequences." *Journal of Black Psychology* 22(2): 1996.

Leigh, Wilhelmina A. *A Health Assessment of Black Americans: A Fact Book.* Washington, D.C.: Joint Center for Political and Economic Studies, 1992.

Milloy, Courtland. "Texaco Tapes a Deep Well of Racism." *Washington Post,* November 10, 1996, Metro Section, p. B1.

Moore Campbell, Bebe. "Black Executives and Corporate Stress." *New York Times Magazine,* December 12, 1982, pp. 37–39, 100–7.

National Center for Health Statistics. *Annual Summary of Births, Deaths, Marriages, Divorces, and Deaths in the United States: 1992.* Table 9. Hyattsville, Md.: National Center for Health Statistics.

National Center for Health Statistics/Centers for Disease Control and Prevention. "National Hospital Ambulatory Medical Care Survey: 1994 Outpatient Department Summary." *Advance Data.* No. 276: U.S. Department of Health and Human Services (June 17, 1996): 1–5.

National Center for Health Statistics/Centers for Disease Control and Prevention. *Suicide Deaths and Rates.* U.S. Department of Health and Human Services, E950–E959, 1991–1994.

Pizzorno, Joseph, N.D. *Total Wellness: Improve Your Health by Understanding the Body's Healing Systems.* Rocklin, Calif.: Prima Publishing, 1996.

"Still Two Americas, Separate, Unequal." *Washington Times,* October 17, 1995, Section A, p. 13.

"Texaco's Telling Tapes." *Washington Post,* November 11, 1996, Section A, p. 28.

U.S. Bureau of the Census. *Current Population Reports: Income, Poverty and Valuation of Noncash Benefits: 1993.* Tables A, G, J, and K. Washington, D.C.: U.S. Government Printing Office, 1994.

U.S. Bureau of the Census. *Current Population Reports. Marital Status and Living Arrangements: March 1975.* Table 1. Washington, D.C.: U.S. Government Printing Office, 1975.

U.S. Bureau of the Census. *Current Population Reports. Marital Status and Living Arrangements: March 1993.* Table 1. Washington, D.C.: U.S. Government Printing Office, 1993.

U.S. Bureau of the Census. *Poverty in the United States: 1992.* Table 9, Series P60–185. Washington, D.C.: U.S. Government Printing Office, 1993.

U.S. Bureau of the Census. *Statistical Abstract of the United States: 1993.* Table 118. On CD-ROM. Washington, D.C.: U.S. Government Printing Office, 1993.

U.S. Bureau of the Census. *Statistical Abstract of the United States: 1993.* Table 732. Washington, D.C.: U.S. Government Printing Office, 1993.

U.S. Bureau of the Census. *Statistical Abstract of the United States: 1994.* 114th ed. Washington, D.C.: 1994. Pp. 138–45.

U.S. Bureau of Labor. Statistics. *Employment and Earnings.* Table 3. Washington, D.C.: January 1994.

U.S. Bureau of Labor. Statistics. *Employment and Earnings.* Table 54. Washington, D.C., 1994.

U.S. Bureau of Labor. Statistics. *Labor Force Statistics Derived from the Current Population Survey: A Databook.* Table C-19. Washington, D.C., 1982.

U.S. Department of Justice. *Bureau of Justice Statistics Bulletin. Prisoners in 1993.* Washington, D.C.: Government Printing Office, 1994.

Villarosa, Linda, ed. *Body & Soul: The Black Women's Guide to Physical Health and Emotional Well-Being.* New York: Harper Perennial, 1994.

Washington, Durthy A. "Conquering Coping Fatigue." *High Technology Careers,* 1996. [Internet]

Whigham-Desir, Marjorie. "Strategies for Coping with Workplace Depression." *Black Enterprise,* September 1993, Vol. 24, No. 2, pp. 77–82.

CHAPTER SIX
HYPERTENSION

Haynes, Karima A. "Why Hypertension Strikes Twice as Many Blacks as Whites." *Ebony,* September 1992, pp. 36–41.

Haywood, Richette L. "Why Black Americans Suffer with More High Blood Pressure than Whites." *Jet,* December 5, 1994, p. 16.

"Heart Disease in African-American Women." American Heart Association, September 17, 1994, pp. 1–3.

Herman, Robin. "Clues in Hypertension Puzzle." *Washington Post,* October 1, 1991.

Knuts-Cheraux, A. W., B.S., M.D., N.D., ed. *Naturae Medicina and Naturopathic Dispensatory.* Yellow Springs, Ohio: Antioch Press, 1953.

Landrine, Hope, and Elizabeth A. Klonoff. "The Schedule of Racist Events: A Measure of Racial Discrimination and a Study of Its Negative Physical and Mental Health Consequences." *Journal of Black Psychology,* 22(2): 1996, pp. 144–68.

Pizzorno, Joseph E., N.D., and Michael T. Murray, N.D. *A Textbook of Natural Medicine.* Seattle: John Bastyr Publications, 1987.

"Social Stress Linked to Hypertension." *Science News,* February 16, 1991, p. 111.

Weiss, Rudolf Fritz. *Herbal Medicine.* Beaconsfield, England: Beaconsfield Publishers Ltd., 1988.

Winslow, Ron. "Blacks Face Higher Risk in Heart Disease." *Wall Street Journal,* March 28, 1996, p. 1.

CHAPTER SEVEN
DIABETES

Dufty, William. *Sugar Blues.* New York: Warner Books, 1975.

Pizzorno, Joseph E., N.D., and Michael T. Murray, N.D. *A Textbook of Natural Medicine.* Seattle: John Bastyr Publications, 1987.

Whitake, Julian M., M.D. *Reversing Diabetes.* New York: Warner Books, 1987.

CHAPTER EIGHT
OBESITY

Knuts-Cheraux, A. W., B.S., M.D., N.D., ed. *Naturae Medicina and Naturopathic Dispensatory.* Yellow Springs, Ohio: Antioch Press, 1953.

"Obesity." *Health Answers.* Applied Medical Informatics, Inc. [Internet]

"Prevalence of Overweight Among Adolescents—United States, 1988–1991." NCHS, Office of Public Affairs. [Internet] MMWR 43(44): 181–221. 1994.

U.S. Department of Health and Human Services. *Physical Activity and the Health of Young People Fact Sheet.* Centers for Disease Control and Prevention/National Center for Chronic Disease Prevention and Health Promotion, March 1997. [Internet]

CHAPTER NINE
ARTHRITIS

Conkling, Winifred. *Natural Remedies for Arthritis.* New York: Dell, 1997.

Knuts-Cheraux, A. W., B.S., M.D., N.D., ed. *Naturae Medicina and Naturopathy Dispensatory.* Yellow Springs, Ohio: Antioch Press, 1953.

Pizzorno, Joseph E., N.D., and Michael T. Murray, N.D. *A Textbook of Natural Medicine.* Seattle: John Bastyr Publications, 1987.

CHAPTER TEN
ADDICTIONS

Griffith, H. Winter, M.D. "Drug Abuse & Addictions." In *Complete Guide to Symptoms, Illness & Surgery.* Los Altos, Calif.: The Body Press, 1996.

Knuts-Cheraux, A. W., B.S., M.D., N.D., ed. *Naturae Medicina and Naturopathy Dispensatory.* Yellow Springs, Ohio: Antioch Press, 1953.

Phelps, Janice Keller, M.D., and Alan E. Nourse, M.D. *The Hidden Addiction and How to Get Free.* New York: Little, Brown, 1986.

Schaef, Anne Wilson. *When Society Becomes an Addict.* San Francisco: HarperSanFrancisco, 1987.

"Trends in the Incidence of Drug Use in the United States, 1919–1992." Substance Abuse and Mental Health Services Administration.

Washington, Linn. "Unjust Crack Cocaine Laws Must Be Repealed." Progressive Media Project, October 1, 1996. [Internet]

CHAPTER ELEVEN
HIV/AIDS

"AIDS & Alternative Medicine: Current State of the Science." Bastyr University, Seattle, Wash. Redmond, Wash: Tree Farm Communications, Inc. Six tapes. Contact: Tree Farm Communications, Inc., 23703 N. 4th St., Redmond, WA 98053.

Lindesmith Center. "Health Emergency: The Spread of Injection-related AIDS Among African Americans." [Internet]

Siano, Nick, and Suzanne Lipsett. *No Time to Wait: A Complete Guide to Treating, Managing, and Living with HIV Infection.* New York: Bantam, 1993.

U.S. Department of Health and Human Services. *HIV/AIDS Surveillance Report.* 8(2), 1996.

CHAPTER TWELVE
CANCER

American Cancer Society. *Basic Facts.* "Racial and Ethnic Patterns." *Cancer Facts & Figures—1997.* [Internet]

Austin, Steve, N.D., and Cathy Hitchcock, M.S.W. *Breast Cancer: What You Should Know (But May Not Be Told) About Prevention, Diagnosis, and Treatment.* Rocklin, Calif.: Prima Publishing, 1994.

Baylor College of Medicine, the M. D. Anderson Cancer Center, the American Cancer Society, and the Robert Wood Johnson Foundation. "NCI Director Says Genetics Minor Factor for Cancer Among Minorities." News Release. Sixth Biennial Symposium on Minorities, the Medically Undeserved & Cancer.

"Cancer Facts." *Cancer Net.* National Cancer Institute. November 1994. [Internet]

Cley, J. William, M.D.; Holly A. Hill, M.D., Ph.D.; Vivien W. Chen, Ph.D., et al. *Journal American Medical Association,* 272: 947–54, 1994.

Michigan Cancer Foundation-Meyer L. Prentis Comprehensive Cancer Center of Metropolitan Detroit. "Original Summaries of Selected CANCERLIT Records Breast Cancer Differences Between African Americans and Caucasians." Information Ventures, 1995. [Internet]

Parker, S. L., T. Tong, S. Bolden, P. A. Wingo. "Cancer Statistics 1997." *CA—A Cancer Journal for Clinicians, 1997;* 47: 5–27.

"Prostate Cancer Among Different Races and Ethnic Groups." *CancerNet.* National Cancer Institute, May 1996. [Internet]

"Reported Cancer Deaths for the 10 Leading Cancer Sites by Race and Ethnicity, United States, 1993." Table 10. Vital Statistics of the United States, 1996. National Institute of Health. [Internet]

Rosenberg, H. M., S. J. Ventura, J. D. Maurer, et al. National Center for Health Statistics. *Births and Deaths, 1995. Monthly Vital Statistics Report, 1996;* 45(3), suppl. 2.

Stephenson, R. A., C. R. Smart, G. P. Mineau, et al. "The Fall in Incidence of Prostate Carcinoma." *Cancer,* 1996; 77; 1342–48.

Swisher, Bill. "Prostate Study Points to Age, Race." Walter Reed Army Medical Center Public Affairs, 1996.

Wingo, P. A., S. Bolden, T. Tong, et al. "Cancer Statistics for African Americans, 1996." *CA—A Cancer Journal for Clinicians, 1996;* 46: 113–25.

INDEX